A CANCER MADE MESS

JESSICA BELL-ALVAREZ

ISBN 978-1-0980-6623-9 (paperback)
ISBN 978-1-0980-6624-6 (digital)

Copyright © 2020 by Jessica Bell-Alvarez

All rights reserved. No part of this publication may be reproduced, distributed, or transmitted in any form or by any means, including photocopying, recording, or other electronic or mechanical methods without the prior written permission of the publisher. For permission requests, solicit the publisher via the address below.

Christian Faith Publishing, Inc.
832 Park Avenue
Meadville, PA 16335
www.christianfaithpublishing.com

Printed in the United States of America

1

The Call

I had finally stopped bleeding for about a week, and the cramps were gone. As I worked in the school office for the summer, I tried putting the distressing events from the last four months out of my mind. However, that attempt was short-lived as more trouble came knocking—or rather, trouble came calling.

On June 21, 2011, I was alone in the office the day I received a call from the doctor that had completed my most recent D and C.

I heard an older man's voice say, "Jessica? This is Dr. Brake."

A bit surprised, I replied, "Oh, hi...yes?" *That's odd*, I thought. *After all the tests I've had, it was always the nurses that called and said the results were fine, not the doctor.*

He continued, "The results of the tissue sample are back. Jessica, the tissue that was taken was cancerous."

Rather than having a million things run through my mind as I would have expected upon receiving such crucial news, I drew a complete blank.

Did he say... All I could manage in response was, "What?"

He started rambling, but all I heard were jumbled phrases.

"...sending off a sample..."
Did he say cancer?
"...results..."
I don't have cancer.
"...wait for a diagnosis..."
It can't be that big of a deal.

"...cancer..."
He said cancer again.
"...refer you to an oncologist..."
Huh? A what-ist? I'm too healthy for cancer.
"...need further treatment..."
Is this some mistake?
"...have to have a hysterectomy..."
A WHAT! That is a mistake for sure.
"...chemotherapy..."
No. This isn't possible.
"...possible radiation..."
Am I in a bad dream? Wake up, Jessi.
"Jessica?"

There was silence. Did I even respond? I don't know. Next thing I knew, he was talking again.
"...get back with you when we receive results..."
I hung up the phone to realize I was in a different room from where I started the conversation. Did I say anything at all? Did I ask any questions? Did we even say goodbye? I don't know. My head was spinning. My life was changed forever with one single phone call.

> *Then the dragon took his stand*
> *on the shore beside the sea.*
> —Revelation 12:18 NLT

2

The Waiting Game

About ten months prior to *the* call, August of 2011, I started having rather bad cramps and heavier bleeding than normal during my menstrual cycle. I thought it was a little odd but didn't think it was much to worry about.

Seven months later, the problem had grown to a point of concern. After a bad break up and moving into my own apartment, I found myself trapped standing in the shower, not being able to get out due to the unbelievable amount of blood gushing down my leg. I stood there several minutes before I was able to slowly get out, as cross-legged as I could manage, trying to slow the blood flow as much as I could. I sat on the toilet and realized there was a stream of blood from the shower to the toilet. As much as I didn't want to see a doctor, I finally decided it was time to go.

The first appointment was with my primary doctor. Drink more fluids. Get rest. Wait for my body to work itself out.

The second appointment was a change of birth control. Then wait for my body to adjust.

On the third appointment, I made it a point to mention that I was having quarter-sized blood clots, but they assured me all was well. Drink more fluids. Get rest. Your hormones are out of whack. Give your body time. More waiting.

Over time, the blood clots grew larger. It felt as if the blood clots were holding back a pool of blood until the pressure became so strong that everything was suddenly released in an unstoppable rush of blood and clots. The rushes of heavy blood flow became more and more frequent and gradually more severe. I made doctor appointments after doctor appointments. No help. I underwent countless pregnancy tests, CTs, blood tests, x-rays, and ultrasounds, yet there were no answers. I was single, living in a studio apartment alone, living paycheck to paycheck while the medical bills were mounting.

Numerous nurses and doctors kept asking how often I had to change my pad. They stated that if I was changing my pad more than once an hour, that was a concern. I tried explaining that a pad wouldn't hold five seconds worth of blood if I was having a gushing moment. I explained that I had to run to a toilet when I felt a rush; otherwise, it got *everywhere*. I'm assuming because I did not tell them the black-and-white answer of, "Yes, I go through more than one pad an hour," they did not think much of the situation. They blew off my answer as an exaggeration.

For most of the tests, there was a one- to two-week waiting period for the results. Waiting was one of the hardest parts. The worry that accompanied not having answers led to an overwhelming feeling of helplessness. I was no longer in control. No matter what I did, I could not influence the speed or outcome of the results. It was out of my hands completely.

One evening, I was having exceptionally bad pains and heavy bleeding. I decided to call Mom for advice. I explained that I felt like I needed to push. She drove the thirty-minute drive to my apartment to take me to the ER. She, along with the many doctors that I had seen, kept assuming that I was having a miscarriage. They gave me probably my fifth pregnancy test and a CT scan to ensure none of my organs had busted. The tests showed I was not pregnant, and all of my organs were fully functional. However, there was a large cyst on my spleen, which was probably from a childhood accident and was not much of a concern since my pain was coming from my "lower right quadrant." Meaning, right above my groin to the right. I heard once again that there was also a lot of "stuff" inside my uterus, which they attributed to my period. In other words, no answers—again.

After waiting on countless tests results, "brush-off" appointments, numerous ER trips, and nonstop bleeding, I had become extremely weak. I continued to go to work, although at times it was difficult. My boss rushed me to the doctor once after almost fainting in her office. The same questions that I had heard countless times before were asked. The most reoccurring ones were, "Are you pregnant?" "Have you ever been pregnant?" "Do you have a chance of being pregnant?"—the answer to all of which was no. No. No. No! I was told to drink more fluids and was referred to a gynecologist across the hallway. I made an appointment for the next week, which was the soonest I could get in. Another week of waiting. Another week of constant bleeding.

At the gynecologist appointment in mid-April, I underwent an ultrasound. The technician looked confused while looking at the screen. I tried to prod the technician for some insight; however, she explained that she was not allowed to give results. That was the doctor's job. The doctor told me too that there was a lot of "stuff" inside my uterus and that my uterine wall was thickened. The doctor casually assured me that there was nothing to worry about. She suggested I wait it out and insisted that things would work themselves out on their own. *How long do I have to wait? I've been waiting!*

A week later, the symptoms had not improved. Unbelievably, they had grown even worse. By this point, I was passing clots the size of my fist, no exaggeration. The rushes of blood flow had become so violent and frequent that I made it a point to not stray far from a bathroom. Luckily at work, my classroom was right next to the bathrooms in the back of the building. When I felt a building pressure, I knew a rush was soon to come. I would go sit on the toilet and push. Blood clots and blood would come gushing out and fill the toilet bowl. Sometimes I didn't make it to the toilet, so I would end up having a large mess to clean up. I felt so frustrated and utterly exhausted. The horrible cramps became exceedingly overwhelming. My mother made the drive to my apartment again after another phone call explaining my symptoms. She immediately rushed me to the ER after seeing the toilet bowl and bathroom floor filled with blood, looking like a murder scene in a horror film.

The ER doctor conducted the same reel of tests and asked the same list of questions—all of which I felt were equally useless and annoying. Another ultrasound. This time, there were two ladies administering the ultrasound. They were both confused and talking about how odd the images were. Mom was there and was able to hear them saying, "That's unusual...look how thick that is," while pointing to the uterus lining. However, yet again I found no answers. I was sent home with the same instructions of getting rest and consuming extra fluids.

At a follow-up appointment with the gynecologist, she asked to see a sample of a blood clot and gave me a small glass vial. I said, "That's not big enough." She looked at me in disbelief but came back with a small jar about the size of a lid off a mouthwash container. *The blood clots won't fit in that either, but if I tell her that, she won't believe me. I guess I can cut off a piece to put in there.*

That evening, when I felt a gush coming on, I took a bowl and sat on the toilet. With one push I filled the bowl with a clot larger than my fist along with the usual enormous amount of blood. No exaggeration. I tore off a piece of the enormous clot and shoved it in the small container.

When I returned to the gynecologist's office the next day, my mother accompanied me. I explained that what I handed them was just a piece of a blood clot, not the whole thing. They didn't seem to believe me. *They think I'm exaggerating. Why won't anyone take me seriously?* The doctor looked me over and stated that she did not see anything abnormal. She ordered another ultrasound. After she reviewed the results, she casually stated that I simply needed to flush some fluids the rest of the evening, and they would try to schedule me for a D and C later that week if I was still having issues.

As I was listening to the doctor explain the plan, I felt another rush building. It was that familiar feeling of, if I were to move, blood would spill everywhere. I knew that if I were to try to explain it to the doctor, she would think it was yet another exaggeration. So, I kept quiet.

After she had left, it was time for me to get dressed. "I can't move," I said to Mom.

She looked confused. "Why?"

"If I move, I'll bleed all over everything," I explained.

She looked irritated and said, "It's about time somebody figured this out, Jessi. Go ahead and bleed all over everything."

That didn't sound like such a good idea to me as I had done that enough. I was tired of cleaning up blood. I decided I would try to hold as much of it as long as I could. While attempting to stand, the pressure became so strong that the flood came bursting through. I couldn't stop it. More huge clots, along with another large amount of blood, gushed all over the table onto the footstool and spilled onto the floor. I closed my eyes in frustration and took a deep breath. When I opened my eyes, I saw what looked like the aftermath of someone being slaughtered on a butcher table. I turned to look at my mother. She was sitting in the chair with a look of utter awe. Her eyes were large. Her mouth was dropped open. She was speechless.

I suddenly felt enraged. *She looks so surprised at something I've been trying to explain and deal with for months now! YES, THIS IS BAD! I KNOW! You're not the one dealing with this.*

While standing there, I stuck my hand between my legs. I gave a good push and caught the huge blood clot that had been holding the flood back. It filled my entire hand, palm, fingers and all. I held it toward Mom and exclaimed, "Look at that! Do you see this? This is what I've been putting up with!"

Mom sat in obvious shock. I felt completely lost and alone. *No one cares to try to figure this out. There is something wrong! This is* not *normal* I felt tears of frustration starting to well up. I told myself, *Crying isn't going to help. Stop it. Get this cleaned up so you can just leave.* With a couple of deep breaths, I fought back the tears and gathered myself.

Realizing I was still holding the awkward blood clot, I asked, "Now what am I supposed to do with this?"

Mom told me to leave it on top of the trash can, not inside, but on top. I grabbed some paper towels and started to clean the examining table off. Mom sat and watched.

I was so lightheaded that I almost fell over when I was trying to wipe off the footstool but luckily caught myself on the wall with my hand, which smeared a grotesque-looking streak of blood on the wall, during which the blood kept rushing. It wouldn't stop. It was everywhere: on the examining table, footstool, wall, trash can, and floor. It did not seem as if cleaning was doing any good; the mess was just getting worse by the second.

Of course, I'm the only one cleaning this. I'm always the only one dealing with this mess. I'm sick of it. No one understands how horrible this is. I'm the only one who is dealing with this crap. I'm the only one dealing with how horrible I feel. I feel so alone.

I heard Mom say, "Jessi, just leave it."

I stopped. She was right. I was doing nothing but making a bigger mess. *I want to go home. I'm not cleaning any more of this. They can deal with it. Have a taste of what I've dealt on a daily basis.*

I threw on my clothes and harshly said, "Let's just *leave*!"

Mom didn't question. She stood up and headed out the door, leaving the mess and huge clot visible for all to see.

As I was walking out of the room, I was so dizzy that I stumbled and fell into the hallway wall. A nurse passed me in the hallway and gave me a questioning side-glance. She went into the room and saw what had to have looked like a murder scene. Before I was at the end of the hallway, the nurse ran out and stopped us, saying, "Hold on! Let me get the doctor." I stopped and leaned against the hallway, glad for the break from walking. Breathing fast and hard, I tried to catch my breath.

The nurse returned, explaining that they were going to do an emergency D and C. *She saw the blood. Someone finally sees how bad it really is. Finally, after four months—finally.* As a rush of relief fell upon me, I suddenly felt very weak at the knees. It must have been noticeable because the next thing I knew, they were offering me a wheelchair to sit in. I was then literately run to another part of the hospital.

They wheeled me to the waiting room before being taken to pre-op. Minutes seemed like hours as we sat and waited. I remember realizing that I was freezing while sitting in the wheelchair, which was an unusual occurrence for me as I was always hot. I started to feel myself become weak, and breathing became harder. Mom watched me turn whiter and whiter until she suddenly stood up, pushed me into a woman's office, and loudly exclaimed, "I need help. My daughter is supposed to be going in for a D and C, and it's been long enough!"

The woman tried to calm her down, but before many words were out of her mouth, Mom exclaimed, "LOOK, LADY! SHE'S BLEEDING TO DEATH!"

The woman took one look at me and immediately grabbed the phone on her desk to tell the other person on the line, "You have to get down here, and I mean *now*." Within ten seconds, I was being wheeled to pre-op. When I stood to get onto the gurney, there was some murmuring between the nurses standing behind me. I asked my mom what was going on, and she told me that they were discussing the pool of blood that was found in the seat of the wheelchair. I was accustomed to seeing blood everywhere; however, that wasn't the case for everyone else. *Good. I'm glad there was a pool of blood. Good. Let them see I'm not lying!*

A slew of different staff came in asking questions, poking, prodding. Things moved very quickly. During the commotion, the anesthesiologist grabbed my hand and told me that he was there for me and me alone, coming in on his day off. He looked at my fingernails. He explained that I was so very low on blood that my nail beds were white because all of my blood was at my essential organs, trying to keep me alive. Had the nurse not stopped me after finding the murder scene in the doctor's room, I would have gone home and bled to death that very day, April 18, 2011.

After hearing that statement, I heard my mother start crying. I will never forget my mother's look of anguish. *Poor Mom, she's so upset. I don't want her to be upset.* She later told me not only was all the blood missing from my fingers, but apparently my lips were as white as a piece of paper.

Next thing I know, I was getting bags of fluids, someone else's blood, and a concoction of other things to be prepped for surgery—all the while I was trying to catch my breath. *Just breathe. They see now. Just breathe.* My mom was still crying as I was being wheeled out of the room and taken to the surgery room. On the way to the D and C, I felt relieved that something was finally being done to help me. For the first time since the ordeal began, I felt someone finally had a small glimpse of what I had been dealing with. I finally felt understood.

After the D and C, my gynecologist met and spoke with my mother, telling her that I was going to be kept overnight for observation. She came in and spoke briefly with me. She said that while administering the D and C, by the time she "got in there," I had stopped bleeding, but she assured me that she "scraped me out very well anyway." As a sidenote, she mentioned some odd grayish grainy substance came out during the procedure but assured me that everything looked normal and that I was fine. Absolutely nothing to worry about, she said. Somehow or another, within an hour of her telling my mother that I was going to spend the night, I was suddenly being dismissed and sent home. I was to come in for a follow-up after the results of the tissue sample were in. More waiting.

Stand firm against him, and be strong in your faith. Remember that your family of believers all over the world is going through the same kind of suffering you are.
—1 Peter 5:9 NLT

3

Ms. Snooty Pants

During the follow-up appointment, my gynecologist told me that the test results showed nothing of any concern. She casually stated that all the tissue samples that were extracted were noncancerous. When I asked about the cause of all the troubles and explained that I was still having light bleeding, she had a condescending air about her that gave the impression that she knew exactly what was wrong and that it was, as she had expressed on several occasions, "no big deal." She explained again, almost seeming annoyed, that I was having problems due to a hormonal imbalance from missing a few birth control pills, and the stress of the breakup was throwing my body off. She had been suggesting that I get Mirena to help balance my hormones before the D and C, but now she was really starting to push the matter.

Not only was my mother strongly against the Mirena, but she made clear of her ill feelings toward my gynecologist. My mother was not impressed with her condescending tone, constant brush-offs, and snooty attitude.

The bleeding continued, getting a little heavier. I made more appointments, each one ending with the same conclusion. Nothing to worry about but with the very strong suggestion of getting the IUD. I eventually agreed to the Mirena after the doctor strongly suggested it several more times. She once again stated that there was no danger in the procedure, and it was the simplest and easiest procedure to solve the problems. It would even out my hormones and stop the bleeding. It would be for the best. *Good. It will be done. No more trouble. Whatever I need to do to make sure this doesn't happen again.*

Unfortunately, after she inserted the IUD a week later, I could feel the strings poking me. I made an appointment to get them clipped. The gynecologist explained that she did not see how they were poking me; they were at the correct length as they were. However, she clipped them to "satisfy me." While there, I explained that my cramping and bleeding were not getting better but slowly growing worse. She once again assured me that was normal too.

Shortly after the appointment, I noticed the strings were still poking me when I would sit down. I was hesitant on calling the doctor. I was worried she would view me as a complainer and a nuisance. After another week of being poked, I finally called to schedule another string-clipping appointment. She once again said that the strings were already short due to the clipping the first time. She explained that I shouldn't be feeling anything.

Her statement made me feel as if she didn't believe that I actually did feel them poking me. Nevertheless, she cut them even shorter and stated that was the shortest they could go. She said it with a tone that told me I was just going to have to deal with it. I asked her again if it was normal for me to still be having severe cramps and now heavy bleeding again several weeks after the insertion of the IUD. She assured me it was perfectly normal. I felt frustrated, thinking, *Well, if I'm going to continue to bleed, then why did I get this stupid thing anyway? I have been on my period for months straight now!*

While sitting at my apartment replaying the last several months in my head, I started to become angry that this was not solved already. Not only was I still in pain and bleeding, but the urge to push had now returned. Out of frustration and sheer desperation, I decided to give it a good, hard to push to see what would happen.

I went to my bathroom, sat on the toilet, and gave several full-on hard pushes. I suddenly felt something large painfully drop inside of me. But strangely, nothing came out. After sitting and evaluating the situation, I noticed the urge to push was gone. *I know I felt something drop, but there's nothing in the toilet besides blood. I don't get it.* I decided to feel around in there to see if I could feel something.

And I did. I felt *something*. About a finger's length inside, there was something large blocking my exploration. I couldn't get past it.

Maybe that's normal? Maybe it's always been there. I can't say I've ever really done this before. I mean, what in the world could it possibly be? It has to be normal.

I contemplated how to tell a doctor what happened when I wasn't even sure myself. Was I imagining things? Did something drop? Did it not? Was *drop* the word? I couldn't quite figure out how to tell my gynecologist and knew that I would get the same, "Oh, you're fine" rigmarole. I decided to avoid feeling like a fool when talking to her and decided to keep the experience to myself.

A month after insertion of the IUD, I went back for the follow-up appointment. On the way to the appointment, I had an eerie feeling that something was about to go wrong. I couldn't explain it, and I really had no clue as to what exactly was going to happen, but I felt something looming in the air above me. Something bad was coming. Accepting there was nothing I could do about it, I tried to ignore the feeling.

The gynecologist arrived in the room followed by a young female student-doctor. The gynecologist wanted the student-doctor to conduct the checkup. I angrily thought, *My doctor isn't even going to be doing this? Of course not. Despite all the crap I've gone through the last few months, she doesn't think my situation is a concern.* The check-up was supposed to be a "one- to two-minute procedure max" (per the gyno), but the student was having difficulties operating the tool and finding the IUD. We all assumed it was because the girl was a student and didn't know what she was doing. With an annoyed glance, the gynecologist swiveled her chair over to the student-doctor to give over the shoulder guidance.

As I lay there being painfully poked and prodded, I couldn't help but glance at my gynecologist and think, *Why can't YOU just do it! I have had enough troubles, and this girl is starting to make me worried, never mind she's HURTING me.* After what seemed an eternity of the student-doctor trying to figure it out, the gynecologist finally took over with the usual cool, calm, and almost snooty attitude.

I was expecting the gynecologist to look at the student-doctor and say, "See, here it is," with her usual condescending tone, but the statement didn't come. She sat there with the tool for a while, trying to find the strings. With a sigh, she explained that she needed to do an exam (with her hand) to find the strings. Seemingly even more annoyed, she explained to the student-teacher that "the patient came in on two different occasions to get the strings clipped. She kept stating it was poking her, so naturally it is harder to locate."

Okay, it's my fault that they are having problems. I should have just dealt with the strings poking me.

Within seconds of the hands-on exam, I noticed a change in her snooty attitude. Something was different.

Is that worry on her face? Ms. Snooty Pants is worried? That can't be good.

> *My heart is troubled and restless.*
> *Days of suffering torment me.*
> —Job 30:27 NLT

4

Frustration

"You have…hmmm," she continued the exam with a confused look on her face.

After a few seconds that seemed like an eternity, she slowly said, "You have…yes. Hmmm…you have a fibroid. A rather large one."

What! A fibroid? As in a…a mass? What are you talking about lady? I don't know what a fibroid is.

While continuing the exam, she said, "And wait…" She pushed further.

"It appears…that you are dilated…wait, let me see."

Huh? How can that be? I felt the rush of the all-too-common sense of worry and confusion engulf my entire body.

"Yes, you are. You are dilated. Dilated to a three," she said in a tone that showed she was as confused as I was.

What? Dilated? Isn't that what women do when they give birth? *I'm not pregnant. I've had tons of pregnancy tests. Too many to count. She knows that. She did a test herself. Right here in this office.*

"You weren't pregnant, were you?" she once again asked the same question that I had been asked countless times before.

Frustration was coming to a head. *No, I WAS NOT, NOR HAVE I EVER BEEN, PREGNANT! No, NO, NO! Everyone keeps asking me that! How many times do I have to take a pregnancy test!* I took a deep breath and responded with irritation, "No, I had lots of tests. You did a test. I'm not pregnant."

"Yes, that's right. We did a test."

Why did I have to remind YOU *of that? Aren't you supposed to be the professional?*

Before I could ask questions, she left the room and took her staff along with her. My mind was reeling. *What if she's wrong? She has been wrong this far. She doesn't really know what she's doing. She was so unconcerned, and now all of a sudden, she knows exactly what is going on? I don't trust her. I don't believe her. I don't like her.*

After at least fifteen minutes of my mind racing, she returned to the room. As I was about to ask some questions, she stated, "At your young age, having a fibroid is rather uncommon. But most likely, the fibroid is nothing to worry about." She then quickly threw in, "However, very rarely, miscarriages can turn into cancer."

There it was. The first time I had heard the *c* word.

But that couldn't be. I have never been pregnant. I have peed on countless sticks, have had over a handful of blood tests to check if I was having a miscarriage. They have done several scans and ultrasounds. How can she say a miscarriage when all the tests have said that's not possible? I know that I was never pregnant, never had a miscarriage—therefore, it can't be cancer. Why would she all of a sudden throw out the cancer *word when my whole situation has been such a nonconcern this entire time? And* NOW *she says cancer? She said the samples she took during the D and C were all fine, not cancerous, so why is she changing her tune now? I don't get it.*

"As for the IUD, it has probably punctured through and is now somewhere in your abdomen. We are going to do an x-ray to locate the IUD." After hearing the news of the fibroid, I had forgotten about the IUD. "If it is, it's a very simple and small procedure to remove it. Just a small incision. It's a quick surgery." She had her "no big deal" air about her again.

How can she be so nonchalant about this? Any part of this! I have been going through hell for months now. Things keep going wrong. No one knows what is going on, her especially. And she's just so casual about all of this while I'm in a living hell.

After the x-ray, they walked me over to the ultrasound room again. During this ultrasound, the ultrasound tech seemed even more uneasy than the ones before. She oddly asked if I was feeling any pressure. *Pressure? Is that what you would call this pain? I don't know!*

I explained that I had been in constant pain for four months and had not stopped bleeding. She shook her head almost as in disgust but kept her mouth shut, as they are trained to do. I didn't bother asking, knowing I wouldn't get any answers.

I returned to the room to sit and wait again, alone with my thoughts. Finally, my doctor came into the room to tell me that she was going to have a nurse call and schedule another D and C with me after she received the results of the x-ray and ultrasound.

I returned to work. I did not want to sit at home and wait for the results. Knowing how the waiting game went, I assumed it would be another week. Surprisingly, the nurse called me later that day to set up another emergency D and C. The image showed that the IUD was dislodged. My doctor wanted to complete another D and C and get it out as soon as possible. I had finally had enough.

No. I am done with her. She obviously has no idea what she is doing. The "fibroid" had obviously been there for the first D and C, and she missed it. She said it showed "nothing." Am I really going to give her another chance? She is trying to rush this, not on my behalf but, rather for hers, trying to fix her errors. I was beyond aggravated. I explained to the nurse that I was going to get a second opinion.

I made an appointment with a gynecologist out of town. The soonest they could get me in was in two weeks. Another wait. During those two weeks, my mind raced more than ever. Not knowing what was wrong was extremely frustrating, irritating, and worrisome. Not having the answers was the scariest experience in my life—up until that point.

*On the hilltop along the road, she
takes her stand at the crossroads.*
—Proverbs 8:2 NLT

5

Good Luck, Jessica

The new doctor had been very specific in stating that he needed *all* of my doctor notes. Tests, procedures, visits, everything they had done—he wanted every detail. I called my old gynecologist's office and asked for my visit notes along with all scans and tests results. They said they would have them ready the next day. The following day, I went in to get them. As the secretary handed over some papers, I asked her if I could also have the results of the ultrasound.

The nurse looked flustered and stuttered around. She mumbled something about not knowing if she could disclose the results.

"I need a copy of it. The new doctor said that he needs it."

She mumbled something and disappeared behind a wall and returned with a second nurse to simply state, "I'm sorry, we're not able to give that to you."

I quickly asked, "Who do I need to talk to, to get them?"

Both nurses looking shocked and stuttered around some more, saying something about not being allowed to give me a copy. I rephrased my question, "Who do I go to, to get a copy of my ultrasound?" My voice level had raised at this point. The same ultrasound tech that had asked me if I was feeling pressure must have overheard because she suddenly appeared out of her ultrasound room, which was two doors behind the front desk.

She loudly asked from behind the two nurses barricading the desk, "Is she wanting the results for her ultrasound?"

I very loudly replied over both of the nurse's heads, "Yes!" The ultrasound tech promptly went into her office. The second nurse literately ran behind the wall again. I looked at the nurse at the desk, and she was looking worried. I gave her a dirty look. *What is your problem anyway? Why don't you want me to get my results?*

The ultrasound technician reappeared carrying a disc. Rather than handing it to the receptionist to hand to me, she rushed out of the door that led behind the desk to personally handed it to me. She gave a look of sympathy and said, "Good luck, Jessica."

Oh no. Good luck, Jessica? It was at that exact moment that I knew something was seriously wrong. *Good luck with what? Does she know something?* Of course, she did. And she could not and would not give any more insight. But I got the cue. Something was wrong. Seriously wrong. I quickly left the office before the other two nurses had the chance to try and stop me.

My mother was just as scared and frustrated as I was on the drive out of town to the new doctor. We were both tired and upset. Despite all the negative feelings, I had a small sense of relief knowing that I was going to a place where I would surely get some real answers. I could feel this was the right call.

The new doctor was an older man. He came into the office with a strong sense of frustration. He said that after reviewing the records I had brought along with me, "the second page of the D and C is missing. The second page is the one with the actual results." He continued to make it clear that he was very upset that the last page was not included in the notes, the most important page. It was honestly nice to see someone else frustrated with what was going on, but I couldn't help but remember the trouble obtaining the disc with the image of the ultrasound. *Why did the nurses leave the most important part of the records off?* I had an eerie feeling it wasn't by mistake, especially considering the amount of trouble I had trying to get that disc. I started to wish I had thought to look over the paper documents to make sure they were all there, but I quickly realized I wouldn't have known what I was looking for.

He put the sonogram that the ultrasound tech personally handed me on display and, with an irritated tone, said, "As you can *clearly* see, you have a large mass in your cervix. It is of significant size. As for the IUD, I have no idea where it is. It could have already come out with all the blood, or it is floating somewhere inside." He grumpily threw in, "I have no idea how they even got the IUD inserted." Finally, someone realized the severity of the situation.

He said that he wanted to get a look at the fibroid. He started the exam and decided to take a sample of it, of me. He pulled out a tool that closely resembled an alligator's mouth. It was a long metal tool filled with razor-sharp teeth on all sides, opening and closing as an alligator's jaw does.

As my mother had always said, I have a high tolerance for pain. I had my fair share of accidents with broken bones and stitches and had handled them all very well. The cramps during the four months prior were bad enough to make me double over. The fist-sized clots I passed were nothing but painful. But when he was pulling pieces of the mass off with the alligator tool, it was a pain I had never experienced before. It was excruciating.

I remember blinding agony as he ripped pieces of the tumor out. He was pulling out pieces of my flesh, of me. Not only was the pain almost completely unbearable, but I could feel it tugging at the innermost part of me. It felt as if he was pulling the most private and personal parts of my insides out. After getting several chunks, he took pity on my moans of agony and finally quit.

He decided he was going to have to do an emergency D and C. *Here we go again*, I thought. I had the option for an ambulance to transport me to the nearest hospital or for us to drive. I chose for us to drive our own and meet the doctor there. On the short trip there, I noticed that the usual cramps were starting again. They would hurt for a few minutes and then subside. *Not again, not now*, I thought. By the time we were in the open lobby area waiting our turn, the pains were so excruciating that I found myself lying on two seats pushed together with my mother kneeling on the floor beside my head, holding my hand through the cramps. I heard her say over and over again, "This is just like labor. These are just like contractions…" It seemed like eternity, but finally about an hour later, I was in the prep room answering the normal overwhelming amount of questions.

Have you had any prior surgeries? Do you have any heart conditions? Do you have a history of any medical conditions? Does your family have a history of any medical conditions? When was the last time you ate? What did you eat? Have you ever been pregnant? Ever had a miscarriage? When was your last menstrual cycle?

The nurse was astonished when I described how I had been on my period for four months straight.

Before I knew it, the D and C was over, and I was in the recovery room talking to the doctor about what he had discovered. He said that what he found was quite unique. He explained that the mass was actually some sort of large tumor that was "hanging" from my uterus by a "string of tissue" down into my cervix. It was like a ball hanging from a string—inside of me.

He explained that it was rare for a person of my age to have a fibroid, let alone at this magnitude, and it was extremely rare that it would be cancerous.

He stated, "I imagine you have had severe pain?"

I said with a sigh of relief, "Yes. Bad." *Finally, someone understands what has been happening!*

He replied "That makes sense because you've been in labor."

"LABOR!" I was baffled. No! *I'm not pregnant!*

He continued, "Your body was trying to pass the tumor, throwing your body into labor. It wasn't able to pass the tumor due to it being connected to your uterine wall by the string of tissue. It's just been hanging in your cervix, and your body has been trying to push it out as a woman's body does during childbirth. Hence, your labor contractions."

I sat in silence, feeling as if things were finally coming together. He must have thought I hadn't understood what he said because he repeated, "You have been in labor for four months. That is why you were dilated and having contractions. The string of tissue was connected to your uterine wall. That, in turn, caused your uterine wall to be irritated, which resulted in continuous bleeding."

I knew that was my answer. I could feel it. When I heard him explain it, I had a sense that I had somehow known that already. It was as if I was experiencing déjà-vu.

That is why I had such a strong urge to push for months. That makes sense. That is why the "cramps" were so severe. They weren't just cramps; they were contractions! For four months! No wonder I felt so exhausted. It is finally figured out and is done. I mean really done this time. No more trouble.

I was going to be able to go home, which I was appreciative of. Oh, and for the IUD? He stated that he found it floating around in my uterus. He got it out.

The nurse who pushed me out of the hospital in the wheelchair was initiating a casual conversation while we waited for my mom to bring the car around. I wasn't much up for talking. I did, however, answer her question as to where I had gotten my previous treatment/care for my condition. When I told her the town, she said, "Ohhhh, I'm sorry. I have heard a lot of negative things about that place." I wasn't surprised. I still couldn't figure out how the old gynecologist missed the fibroid in my uterus in the first place—and then those darn test results. Why was everything so difficult?

I told Mom in the car, "That's what is really happening to me, Mom. I just feel it. He's got it right. That's it. It's finally figured out."

> *They were gripped with terror and writhed in pain like a woman in labor.*
> —Psalm 48:6 NLT

6

Sharing the News

After receiving the life-altering phone call diagnosing me with not only a disease but what seemed as an end-of-life sentence, I sat in silence. I'm not sure how long I sat there. Before I knew it, the clock was nearing the end of the workday. I decided I had better call Mom and let her know.

As I was dialing Mom, I was contemplating how I was going to tell her. The phone rang and rang again. Oblivious to what had happened hours earlier, she happily answered, "Hello?"

I didn't know how to say something I didn't understand myself yet. I felt as though I was having an out-of-body experience. *Start off easy…*

"Dr. Brake called back," I said.

"Yeah?" Her tone had changed from light and airy to hard and serious.

How do I say this? How can I say something that doesn't seem real? I sat silent. She impatiently prodded, "*And?*"

It came out of my mouth as though someone else was speaking for me, "He said that the fibroid was cancerous."

Hearing my own voice say those words felt so surreal. We sat in silence.

I heard her begin to cry.

Sobbing, she said, "We will handle this. We will get through this."

She's crying. It can't be that bad. It can't be that big of a deal. And what does she mean get through this? Get through what? I have to get through this? What is there to get through? Getting through means there's another side. That other side is so far away—this side is so far away. What side am I on? Where am I?

Hearing my mother's distress continue gave me a quick glimpse of how serious the situation was. I felt panic creeping up on me. It was almost there. I swallowed hard. *No. Keep it together.* I quickly got off the phone. She threw in a distressed "I love you" rather than the normal quick, happy "I love you." *She's acting as if this is the last time she is going to talk to me. Does she think I'm going to die? Am I going to die?*

I did not tell anyone else that day. I finished my day at work and returned to my apartment to be alone. I called no one, and no one called me. I felt so far away from everything I had ever known. I spent the evening feeling as if I was in another dimension. I was lost somewhere in the darkness—lost, alone, confused, stranded—darkness, fear.

Just hours ago, everything was fine. What happened to yesterday? I was fine yesterday. How can things change so quickly? I can't believe this is happening to me. To me. I am too young for cancer. I feel fine now. The problems were supposed to be over. Is this real?

I spent the night sleepless, lost in thoughts.

Cancer. The word haunted me. It was looming over me. Something I could not grasp. Could not understand. Unreal.

Cancer. Cancer. Cancer. Cancer? Me? Die? Dying? Dead? Death?

I turned inward. I pulled all of it in. All the emotions, thoughts, worries, fear. All of them were mine. They were overwhelming. Too overwhelming. By the time morning had arrived, I still hadn't grasped the concept that I had a life-altering moment.

I went to work to try to get a sense of normalcy. My mother called. The first thing she told me was how she had shared the news with my family, another state away.

"What? You told them?" I exclaimed. The thought of telling family members honestly hadn't even crossed my mind. I needed some time to process what happened before I could deal with explaining what happened to anyone else. I didn't know what was happening. I didn't feel comfortable with anyone else knowing something I hadn't yet grasped.

Mom retorted, "Well, Jessi, they would have to find out at some point, and Mom would kill me if she knew I hadn't told her." I suppose it was something that needed to be done, yet that was the last thing on my mind.

Within the next few days, my grandmother, whom I am very close to, was rushed to the hospital. My grandmother and I have a special bond. She lived next door while I was growing up, and I always viewed her as an additional mother. It was well known that when her stress level became high, she had heart problems. *I'm the reason she's in the hospital.* I started to feel angry with myself.

When I called the hospital to get a hold of my grandmother, she told me, "You take care of yourself, you hear?" I could hear the stress and worry in her shaky voice. I think she was crying. I had never seen or heard my grandmother cry before. She was the toughest lady I had ever known.

I responded, "No, Grandma, you take care of yourself. You're the one in the hospital. I'm going to be fine." *I don't feel fine, but I don't want her to know that. I am the strong one. Don't let her see how worried you are, Jessi.*

Over the next few days, the process of realizing what happened hadn't progressed much further. I was still in shock. From what I knew of cancer, it was a death sentence, for older people. I kept asking myself how something like that could happen to me. A young healthy woman diagnosed with cancer? I knew no one my age that had been diagnosed with cancer.

I kept having flashbacks to visiting my aunt Joyce who eventually succumbed to the cancer. She had been diagnosed with breast cancer that spread to her brain. She was at home, in a hospital bed, looking frail and weak the last time I saw her. I could tell it took all of her effort to just smile and say hi. Seeing the effect it had on my cousin Megan that her mother was passing was heartbreaking. To hear that Megan had passed in a car wreck not too long after Joyce had passed was even more earth-shattering. Was that what was going to happen to me and my immediate family? Was I going to die on a hospital bed, followed by my family falling apart?

The thought of dying, leaving my family, hurting my family, losing my future was too much to handle. When I would think of those things, I could feel an overwhelming feeling of panic starting to build deep inside of me. I was afraid to let it out, afraid that I wouldn't be able to get it back under control if it were to overcome me. I needed to be calm. I needed to keep it together. I didn't know what was happening and couldn't afford to lose my mind in a whirlwind of emotions.

Over the next few days, questions started coming. Not from me but from my family. "He said you have cancer?" "Do you still have cancer, or was it taken out?" "What do they want to do?" "He said hysterectomy?" "Did he say what doctor he was referring you to?" When are they going to refer you?" "What kind of cancer?" "What exactly did he say?" "Did he say when the results would be back?"

This is too much. I can't handle all of this. Too much, too soon. I don't have answers. I don't even have a realization of what happened yet, let alone any answers to the hundreds of questions you just asked me.

They kept asking every day. New questions. I was annoyed. I had no answers, yet they expected me to have a wealth of information. I knew nothing. I knew absolutely nothing. At that point, I wasn't even sure if I could tell someone my birth date, let alone details about a phone call I barely understood. I felt frustrated and aggravated that they expected me to know the answers. Personally, I didn't want to think about it. I wanted to avoid it. I was firmly planted in denial and wanted to stay there.

After about a week, I got tired of the nonstop questions, so I finally called the doctor to get some answers to get them off my case. I talked to the nurse. "Your results are not in yet." I transferred the message on back to home base.

How long will it be until the results are in? Did you ask what doctor they are referring you to? Do you have to have the hysterectomy? Or the chemotherapy? Or the radiation? This made me even more frustrated. I thought, *No, I did not ask the reel of questions you have for me daily! I DO NOT KNOW!*

After another couple of days of receiving the same third degree, I called again out of frustration. The nurse said the same thing as before: "Your results are not in yet." *Great, I have to deal with the same reel of questions again. This is frustrating. Just give me some answers.* After asking some questions, I found out that they were waiting for the results to say what type of cancer I had so that they could then refer me to an oncologist. *So I have to wait to see what type I have before they can refer me.* The nurse had no additional answers. However, I managed to get the number for the place that was testing my sample.

I called the number and discovered that I was talking to a receptionist for a large hospital. I tried explaining briefly my situation and asked to speak to the people who were testing cancer samples. She did not know whom to send me to. She acted as if it was her first day and as if the place was not known for testing samples. I recall yelling at her out of frustration. She responded with sympathy; that amplified the feeling of helplessness. There was nothing I could do. It was just a waiting game. Another waiting game.

After telling the family of the no news, it was the same response from the family, just intensified. The questions had become more stressed, more critical, more frustrated. It was the same response from me, yet with intensified feelings. "I don't know. I tried. I don't know. I know nothing! I can't get any answers! I tried!"

What do they expect me to do! I have no answers! I tried to find out what was wrong! I tried! I tried calling, and I talked to some dumb lady that did not know anything! I DON'T KNOW! If they want to know so badly, why don't they call? I have done all that I can do. Why am I the only one having to deal with this? Why can't they pitch in? I can't do this.

After another week of waiting, my twenty-fifth birthday came and passed. Not much of a celebration. Went to lunch with a friend and her daughter. Went home to my apartment to be with my cat. I spent the night sleepless, wondering if this was the last birthday I was ever going to have.

Three weeks after having the cancerous fibroid removed, I called the doctor for a third time and asked to talk to the doctor himself. I asked him if I would need a hysterectomy. He abruptly replied, "Yes.

You will need further treatment: a hysterectomy and possible chemotherapy and radiation."

He then said that he would just go ahead and refer me to an oncologist now rather than wait for results. I would be seeing a female oncologist that he highly recommended in Kansas City, two hours away from where I lived. Her nurse would be calling me to set up an appointment.

I told the family, expecting them to finally be satisfied with some answers. Instead, they retorted with a new reel of questions. "How does he know you need the hysterectomy?" "What's the oncologist's name?" "Did he say when they will call you?" "How soon will you get in for the appointment?" *I DON'T KNOW! WHY DIDN'T YOU CALL!*

The answer of, "Yes, I would need a hysterectomy," did have a huge impact on the vision of what I wanted my life to look like. I was not going to be able to have children. I loved children. I was a preschool teacher. Unconsciously realizing I had a very long journey ahead of me, I did not have time or the ability to suffer that loss at the moment. I continued to push down the feelings. Every once in a while, they would try coming up to overwhelm me, but I would quickly push them back down.

I finally told my coworkers. One of them started crying and gave me a hug. I felt as though I should probably cry, so I cried for about twenty seconds. It felt almost fake. Disconnected. Not real. Nothing felt real anymore. Not even crying.

The oncologist's nurse called me to set up a date. She stated that the doctor that he recommended had too many patients, so I would be seeing a different doctor. That worried me. *Will I not get as good of care? It's a guy, so how will he understand how I feel about not having children? Am I getting second best? The appointment is over a week away. Why does everything have to take so long? I hate these waiting games.*

In the time it took for the oncologist appointment to roll around, the realization that I had cancer started to seep in. In turn, I continued to pull myself into my deep, dark hole—losing sleep, not eating, cutting off talking to people. When it was mentioned, I acted cool, calm, and collected, as if it didn't bother me. I told myself that it didn't really bother me. I put up a wall so that the realization could not soak in any further. I had to keep it together.

> *I am on the verge of a collapse,*
> *facing constant pain.*
> —Psalms 8:17 NLT

7

Johnson

The thirty-minute drive to my mother's house was a blur. Before I knew it, I was pulling into her driveway in a daze. We got in her car and headed toward Kansas City to the University of Kansas Cancer Center in Overland Park.

It was a quiet and dreary two-hour drive. Mom was nervous, I could tell. I told myself, *She's always nervous when driving somewhere new.*

When we arrived to our destination, I noticed the building was huge. We met my sister in the parking garage and found our way through the many hallways to a large waiting room. Two very busy women were sitting behind the front desk, shuffling tall stacks of paper. *What do I do? Do I go up to the desk?* I looked back to Mom and Laveda for guidance; they were standing behind me, chatting among themselves.

I slowly approached the desk and nervously said, "I'm here for an appointment." One of the ladies glanced up with a smile and asked me to fill out a check-in sheet. After she read my name, she started riffling through a basket of papers to find a set stapled together with my name on it. She gave me a clipboard stuffed full of forms and directed me to have a seat while filling them out.

I headed straight to the first set of three open chairs I could find. I didn't sit in the middle; I didn't want to be in the middle of anything. I didn't want any of this to be about me. Mom and Laveda sat beside me, still chattering away while I started to fill out the paperwork. I noticed my hand was shaking. Hoping no one noticed, I wrote faster in an attempt to hide the trembles.

As I was flying through the stack of paperwork, I came to a section labeled "current or past ailments." As I was quickly checking no to all the listed ailments, I came to an immediate halt when I read the word *cancer*.

Cancer?

I sat and stared at the box. *Do I really have to check that little box? I've never had to check any of these, and now I'm supposed to check that one? The worst one?* I skipped box. After completing the rest of the paperwork, I returned to stare again at the little box.

How can a simple little box hold such tremendous meaning? For the rest of my life, I will have to mark that box. I will never be able to fill one of these out again without checking that little box that says cancer. *My life is changing forever, right now, this very moment. I will never be the same.*

Taking in the moment, I slowly started to look around the room.

Sitting to my left was an extremely skinny man with a blue sling mask over his nose and mouth coughing profusely. Sitting to my right was a pale and tired-looking woman with a navy stocking cap. When I noticed she did not have any hair at the nape of her neck, I realized she was bald. A nurse was pushing an older pale bald gentleman in a wheelchair. He had tubes coming out of the neck of his shirt connecting to a bag at the back of his wheelchair.

I was suddenly stricken with complete and utter fear. *These people have cancer.* The realization hit me like a ton of bricks.

I don't belong here. All of these people are old—old and sick. I'm not old. I'm not sick. I'm sitting among pale skinny walking skeletons that look like they are barely clinging to life, and I don't belong here. I feel like I'm in the land of the dead. I do NOT *belong here. I'm in some nightmare where there is death all around me, trying to drag me down with it. I'm too young to be here. Look at all of these old sick people. I'm not sick. Wake up, Jessi, wake up!*

I gave myself a pinch on the arm, thinking the pain might refocus me on something other than the fear, but it did not help. I pinched again, even harder; however, compared to the chaos I was feeling inside, my mind barely noticed the pain from the pinch. I was terrified. Completely and utterly terrified.

I looked at my mother and sister, who were still chattering away. *I want to leave. Can I just not mark the box? But if I don't mark the box, they are going to wonder what I am doing here. I have to mark the box.*

As I slowly placed my first check mark in "that box," I felt something change inside of me. It was as if it was finalized. I had cancer.

Am I really going to become one those? A cancer patient? Am I going to be pushed around bald with tubes and a mask? Am I going to be sick like that? Am I going to become a walking skeleton?

It was almost too much to bear, but I realized I couldn't break down right there, right then. *Get it together. Stop. Stop. Stop it. Don't you cry. Stop it. Not here. Not now.* After deciding to *just make it through this appointment*, I managed to push down the feelings.

As I kept looking around, I realized there were no smiles in the room. There was no laughter. There were hushed voices and distressed faces. Then I heard it. My mother and sister had started to giggle. I glanced over to hear a brief part of their conversation. *I'm facing the realm of death, and you guys are sitting there giggling about frozen hot dogs. Do they really have no idea what is going on here?*

I decided to keep to myself and returned to looking at the room of death. They then tried to get me to join in on their lightheartedness. I shot them an evil look and returned to my despair. They got the hint and became silent. *Finally. They shut up. This isn't fun for me. This isn't a social gathering for me. This is life or death. And it's looking more like death to me.*

Directly in front of me was an older couple sitting beside each other, staring at the floor, appearing completely disconnected from each other, each lost in their own thoughts. Their arms were touching, yet they were obviously so out of touch to each other. I couldn't help but feel the same. Disconnected. Misunderstood. Alone.

When a nurse appeared and called my name, I followed her through yet another array of hallways, rooms, doctors, and walking skeletons.

They asked my name and date of birth. I stuttered around, trying to remember my birthday. They then placed a wristband on my arm. It was the same wristband that all the sick people in the waiting room were wearing. Looking down at the band, I realized I was just labeled a cancer patient.

They placed us in a room with no sink, no instruments, and no examining table. There were just big comfortable chairs and a small table. *What an odd room to see a doctor in. What kind of doctor am I seeing? A doctor room without an examining table?*

We waited. And waited. It seemed an eternity. During this time, my mind continued its usual banter. Relentlessly. *This bracelet means I have cancer. I've been labeled a cancer patient. I'm one of those people in the waiting room. Is this really happening? Why is this happening? What am I going to do now? How am I going to make it through this? Am I going to die?* My mind would answer with, *Just get through the appointment so you can go back home where nothing is wrong.*

Then we heard a ruckus outside our door. There was a man's voice noticeably upset. "Her records are gone. They don't have any record of her. Her records are gone." Were they talking about me? Were they referring to that missing page on the D and C results?

Finally, a short, slender older man came in and introduced himself as Dr. Johnson. He brought chairs and some other doctors along with him. He started off by stating that he remembered when he was twenty-five and how he could not have imagined how such an event would have "turned his world upside down." *Yes, that is how I feel. Okay. I am going to like him.* He went on to explain that when my most recent D and C was completed, it was determined that I had uterine sarcoma. A cancer of the uterine wall itself. It was a rare type of cancer, and it was most likely reoccurring—meaning, it would probably come back. *Oh God, I'm dead. I'm going to die. Cancer is going to kill me. My life is over. It's going to come back until it kills me.*

After a very long and intense conversation, we were headed to a different room with an actual examining table. While sitting there waiting for the doctor to arrive to do the exam, Mom started crying. It hurt me so bad to see her crying. I had seen her cry maybe a handful of times in my life, and now she was crying because of me. I knew she thought I was going to die. I did not want her to have those thoughts, nor could I handle seeing her like that. I was barely able to handle my own feelings, let alone someone else's. I couldn't handle it.

Very coldly, I said, "Mom, just leave if you're going to cry."

Looking insulted, she stormed out of the room. My sister proceeded to inform me that I was being mean to Mom and that she just loves me and has a right to cry. Instead of agreeing, I snapped back at my sister, "I can't handle her crying right now. I'm trying to deal with all of this, and I can't handle her crying. There's too much. I just can't. If you're going to hound me about it, you can leave too."

My sister decided it was a waste of air to argue with me and stood silent. The doctor completed the exam, and we were taken back to the "comfy chair" room. Reunited with Mom, I saw that she still looked flushed, as though she had been crying during the entire exam. She sat silent, looking forward, not making eye contact with me, obviously very mad with me. *I don't really care if she's mad. I've got too much I'm dealing with on my OWN.*

(I did not find this out until about a year after this took place, but when Mom left the room, she went back to the "comfy chair" room where she met with the onsite psychologist. The psychologist told her, "She told you to leave because she thinks you're thinking she's going to die. She couldn't handle anyone having those thoughts. She's scared she's going to die." Psychologists have a funny way of reading minds.)

While waiting for the doctor to come back into the room, a nurse gave me what I assumed was a depression test—questions about whether I was feeling sad, thinking of death, change of appetite, weight loss, sleeping more, disconnection from other people, among other questions. Before I knew it, I had answered all the questions with a yes. Glancing at the sheet, I realized I had the highest score possible. I contemplated changing the answers, but I thought, *Oh well, who cares? Let them know the truth.*

Next thing I knew, an entire team of psychologists were in there talking to me. I calmly and casually admitted to the dreadful answers, yet I repeatedly answered that I didn't need to talk about it.

Next thing I knew, I had two new prescriptions. I didn't care to pay attention to what they were.

The doctor returned and informed us that I did indeed need a hysterectomy and discussed what that was going to look like. He drew a lot of odd-looking pictures and used a lot of medical jargon that I did not understand. He then explained that, yes, I would also need chemotherapy. He was very concerned with the amount of weight I had recently lost: fifteen pounds in a few weeks was not healthy. He prescribed me a medication to help me eat and gain weight, explaining that chemotherapy patients do best when they do not lose weight.

My sister very diligently took notes in the corner of the room. Now looking back, I wish I would have recorded our conversation due to all the confusion we had after the appointment. "He said this ——" "No, I heard this ——" "No, I thought he said this——" Although the notes did help immensely, three sets of ears led to three significantly different versions.

Be on guard. Stand firm in the faith.
Be courageous. Be strong.
—1 Corinthians 16:13 NLT

8

Downhill

After that appointment, things started their descent downhill. Actually, it was just me that went downhill. I am not proud of this time period in my life. However, I am writing it truthfully in hopes of finding someone who is in the midst of the same mistakes I made, to reach them and show them there is a way out.

Hearing that the cancer was most likely reoccurring kept repeating in my thoughts. My mind suddenly turned into a movie reel showing my death. It kept playing scenes of me dying. Dying on a bed at home. Dying in a hospital. Slowly withering away. Complete loss of control. I was terrified. Lost. I felt alone, in a whirlwind. I was dying. So young. I couldn't talk about it. I couldn't think about it. I couldn't face it. My mind was stuck in a negative cycle, leading to negative actions and, hence, a negative life.

Maybe I subconsciously decided I was going to die so I thought, *Who cares anyway?* Maybe I was wanting to go ahead and die now to spare the hassle of dying of cancer. Or maybe it was because of the simple fact that dying was too scary and too hard to think about, so I found a distraction. Or it could have quite possibly been a combination of all the above. For whatever reason, I started hanging out with a new crowd.

The careless crowd. Each member in the crowd obviously had some issues of their own, but no one talked about them. No one asked. I was accepted as a newcomer without questions. Everyone there was there to simply avoid their own lives. Each there for their own hidden reasons.

We found random things to do, places to go. Bars, house parties, concerts, out-of-town trips, swimming in local lakes—anything to avoid reality. We never did any drugs, or maybe I should say, *I* never did any drugs. I honestly can't say what everyone else was doing. But for me, it was just liquor, hard liquor. It didn't matter if it was a weekend or a weekday; the drinking continued. Late nights. Early starts. Somehow I managed to make it to work every day, hungover, but nonetheless there—teaching preschool. A hungover preschool teacher might be hard to imagine, but that was me. As embarrassed and ashamed as I was of my actions, it didn't stop them. We stayed out late and drank too much. On weekends, we would start taking shots of hard liquor the next morning at 9:00 a.m. just to spend the entire day drunk and do it all over again.

I stopped answering calls from the people who actually cared about me. It was easier to push down any feelings that I had while I was hanging around the people who didn't know the truth. To avoid the fear. Avoid the truth.

It was no surprise the majority of the crowd had lost their driver's license after being caught drinking and driving too many times. That did not necessarily stop them from driving, however. Soon I picked up on the carelessness and started driving—drunk. Even after witnessing a fatal car accident where a drunk driver ran a stop sign and killed two young girls in my front yard a few years earlier, I still drove intoxicated countless times. I knew better. Being so irresponsible, I recklessly took for granted the one thing I was terrified of losing—life itself.

> *Then Jesus said to the woman, "I was sent only to help God's lost sheep—the people of Israel."*
> —Mathew 15:24 NLT

9

Surrogacy

Considering my young age and the fact that I did not have any children of my own, my oncologist suggested that I meet with a doctor who specializes in preserving eggs and ovaries. They scheduled the appointment for me, so I agreed to go. I had thought the nurse told me my appointment was at four o'clock.

When Mom and I arrived at 3:45 p.m., I couldn't help but notice the disgusted look from the nurse at check-in. I wondered what that was about but figured she was in a bad mood. We ended up sitting in the waiting room until five thirty, watching nurses walk out of the office, closing for the day, shooting me dirty glances on their way out. Finally, a very disgruntled nurse called my name. She led me to a room with the doctor already in it. I remember thinking once again, *Wow that's unusual. The doctor is waiting on me?*

The doctor did not hesitate in telling me that my appointment was at noon and that it was now closing time. Normally, I would have been gushing out apologies, feeling horrible for being an inconvenience. He sat and stared at me. I suppose he wanted me to apologize, give some hint of remorse, or even simply care. I, in fact, did not care. With feeling as if my life was ending, the last thing I cared about was whether or not I was an inconvenience to someone. My consideration for other people had left, very unlike the normal me. I simply looked at him with a blank face. He was obviously irritated when I casually said, "Oh, I thought they told me four o'clock."

He took a deep sigh. This meeting was not off to a good start.

He took me into his office and started discussing my options—or actually, lack of options. He explained that I might be able to opt for my ovaries to be frozen. It would cost an unbelievable amount of money every year to keep them frozen, money I didn't have. It was like paying rent for a place for my ovaries to stay in a freezer. He then also informed me that if the cancer had spread to my ovaries, then they would not be able to do anything for me—at all. The "bad news" actually didn't really bother me at the time.

I'm not sure if it was the fact that I did not want someone else carrying my baby, or the fact that I was upset to have to pay someone to hold on to something that I didn't want to give up, or that I simply did not care, but I chose to pass on the option to have my ovaries frozen. He made it a point to tell me that this was a once-and-done decision. If I decided I didn't want to save the eggs, there was no going back. Ever. I told him I did not want to save the eggs.

At the time, I could not imagine having someone else carry *my* precious child. The idea of someone else having control of its life when I could not do it myself was unbearable. I did not want to be in the situation I was in the first place, and having to make a major decision that could potentially affect the rest of my life was not something I was willing to participate in. At one point, I remember thinking, *What's the point if I'm going to die anyway?*

My family and friends very gently hinted that I may want to consider it more.

"After you make this decision, there is no turning back."

"If you adopt, someone will have carried that baby, just like if you had a surrogate, but this one would actually be yours."

"It would be worth a shot, just in case you change your mind later. You would have that option."

Yes, those were good points, but my mind was set.

Looking back, of course, I wish I would have said yes, save my ovaries. There is no price on having a child of your own. It's priceless. However, I was not in the right frame of mind to make lifelong decisions when I wasn't sure I was going to have a life to live. But I believe God influenced my decision for a reason. Had I set my mind on saving the eggs, had I set my mind on having a chance to hold, raise, and cherish a child of my own flesh and blood, had I had my heart set on the possibility of a bright future with a child of my own, I would have been crushed to later find out that the cancer had already spread to both of my ovaries.

> *But as for me, I almost lost my footing. My feet were slipping, and I was almost gone.*
> —Psalms 73:2 NLT

10

Stranger in the Dark

During of one of my unfortunate drunken escapades, the group I was with decided to go swimming in a pool out of town that belonged to friends of a friend. I had always loved swimming, and I had no idea whose house it was. *Perfect.* I didn't want to be around the people who really knew me. Avoiding all familiarity was my ultimate goal.

I don't remember who drove. Not having bathing suits didn't matter. It was dark, and we all swam in our underwear. When it was time to go, one of the other girls couldn't find her shirt. After several minutes stammering around searching, the other people were growing impatient. She grabbed a hand towel, haphazardly tried to cover what she could, and we headed back to the car.

We walked past a group of apparently sober strangers sitting on some concrete steps. As I was hoping to pass unnoticed, I realized how nearly impossible that was. After all, I was following a topless girl. I could feel the judging eyes on our group as we passed. I put my head down and tried to hurry along in my drunken haze. Just as we had put our backs to them, I heard someone say, "Jessi!" I stopped cold in my tracks. Someone sitting on the steps had just said my name.

This was supposed to be the group of people that I had no other ties to. This was supposed to be a safe place to pull my "unsafe antics." To be stupid without anyone knowing. I turned around to face them. I was so drunk I could barely stand straight. *Act sober, just act sober.* I squinted, trying to figure out which stranger had said my name.

"Jessi Bell?" he said again, almost in disgust.

How does he know my last name? Oh no.

I felt embarrassed. Embarrassed that I was in the situation I was in, embarrassed that I was drunk, embarrassed that I didn't know who obviously knew me so well. The alcohol was clouding my vision and my thinking. I looked back to see if someone else in my group might save me and start talking. They were gone, already lost in the dark, on their way to the car. *Oh no, they left me. I don't remember where we parked.*

I turned back around to look at the stranger and tried to play it off with a casual, "Oh, hi." I still couldn't quite see his face in the darken drunk haze. I suddenly felt a dizzying swoosh come upon me and stumbled. I grabbed the side of the pool for balance.

He responded with, "Wow... I'm surprised to see *you* here."

That's it. I'm busted. I stood quiet for a moment, trying to gather myself, trying to analyze the situation I had somehow got myself into.

It was someone who knew me very well. Knew the responsible me. Knew the Jessi who would never do anything dangerous or dumb or hang with the wrong crowd. The Jessi that didn't stay out past dark. Yet there I was, stumbling around trying to follow a topless girl at two or three in the morning at some stranger's house and now, most likely, lost.

At that very moment, someone grabbed my arm and said, "Come on, let's go." It was one of people from the group I was with. They had come back for me. A wave of relief rushed over me as they led me back to the car. I looked back and caught one last time glimpse of who knew me so well before rounding the corner.

His face was familiar. Very familiar. But I couldn't quite place who it was. *I know I would know who it was if I wasn't so drunk right now.* It was someone I knew well. *But who was it?* I couldn't quite put my finger on it. To this day, I still can't place who the stranger in the dark was. But that stranger brought back a small sense of reality during a time I was doing all that I could to escape it. The run-in served as a reminder that I was still Jessi. Despite what I was going through, it was still me. No matter how hard I tried to forget what was really happening in my life, to forget the horrible diagnosis, to forget the insurmountable odds I was facing, to forget the life that I had that was being ripped away from me, it was still there—following me, even in the darkness.

> *You, L*ORD*, keep my lamp burning; my*
> *God turns my darkness into light.*
> *—Psalm 18:28 NIV*

11

Hysterectomy

The day had finally come, July 18, 2011. My mom and I drove the two-hour drive in silence yet again. We met my sister at the hospital and checked in. They were both very obviously worried, almost frantic. I, on the other hand, was somehow eerily calm. Everyone else around me seemed to understand the seriousness of the matter, but all I felt was numbness. It was not sinking in that this was one of the most important days in my life, if not the most important.

This surgery was going to determine whether or not my cancer had spread and in turn "seal my fate." If the cancer spread beyond the uterus, I was going to die. If the doctor did something wrong, I could die. If he missed one cell of cancer, I could die. Never once did any of these thoughts cross my mind, although I'm positive it pounded my sister's and mother's minds relentlessly. I was in shock, not able to think clearly. I was numb. My mother's friend whom she had not seen in years came in from another state. Mom made a loud yell and jumped up and ran to her when she saw her. They started crying and laughing. I sat in silence as the two played catch up.

It seemed the hour long wait flew by in a blink. Suddenly my name was being called by a nurse. *It's already my turn? That was fast. I did not even get enough time to think about this yet.*

Suddenly my mother stopped talking to her friend and looked at me with tears in her eyes. She gave me a big hug and told me how much she loved me. I stood there in shock. My sister came up to me, crying, and told me she loved me. I felt a rush of panic when I realized they were saying their last goodbyes, as if I was going to die.

Why are they talking to me like I'm going to die? Should I be worried? I don't want to die. They think I'm going to die. Just calm down. You have to do this. You have no choice.

As I followed the nurse out of the room, I answered her reel of questions absentmindedly. I was suddenly numb again. I was numb up until the point I woke up and tried opening my eyes. I tried moving around and felt a gagging feeling in my throat.

I remember someone saying, "Jessica, just relax," in an anxious tone. They sounded worried. *What's wrong? Where am I? What's going on?* "Jessica wait, just wait..."

I started gagging. They started yelling, "All right! Okay!" and suddenly pulled something large out of my throat and chest. I took a gasp of air and blacked out.

It seemed within seconds I heard someone say, "Breathe! Come on, breathe!" I woke up in the recovery room in extreme pain. I had thought the alligator-teeth tool was painful. Whoa, that was nothing. I kept telling the nurse that I was hurting. She told me, "Honey, I have given you all that I can. You stopped breathing on us because we gave you too much."

If she gave me pain medicine, why am I hurting so bad? This is unbearable. She finally gave me more. The pain faded, and I blacked out again. She woke me up, telling me, "Breathe, Jessica." I would take a gasp of air and black back out. The poor nurse had to tell me with every breath to breathe. I'm not for sure how much time passed until I was breathing on my own without reminders. With that, the pain returned. She wouldn't give me more this time. I couldn't bear it. I felt every inch of my flesh that was cut by the knife. In and out of consciousness I started to pray, *Please, God, help me!* The nurse immediately went to get the doctor.

They placed an epidural in my spine. *Finally, oh, finally* the pain subsided. Next thing I knew, my mother and sister were with me in the recovery room, crying and smiling at me. I told them that the nurse saved my life. They continued talking and brushed over my comment as if it was the anesthesia talking. I became irritated when I noticed they did not quite understand the gravity of the situation.

I snapped at them, "She saved my life! She had to tell me to breathe with every breath!"

It was then that they both lost their smiles, and I insisted that they write down her name, and we get her something special. My sister wrote down her name.

After explaining what had happened and talking with the nurse, it was decided that I had a high tolerance for pain medicine and anesthesia. My mom assured me that it would soon be over, and I would be up in my room, asleep.

A couple of hours later, I was finally in my room, but still not asleep. The pharmacy had not sent up my needed medicine, so the beeper on my drip bag kept going off because it was low. It would give an abrupt and very loud BEEP, BEEP, it seemed like every ten seconds. After a few minutes, the nurse came in to turn off the beep thankfully. I was in the midst of my sorrow when BEEP, BEEP—again. By this time, I was quite annoyed and too medicated to understand what it was. It continued on for several minutes, which seemed an eternity. I couldn't handle it anymore. It was driving me *nuts*. I was drugged, tired, in pain, mad at the world, and there was something annoyingly beeping at me, keeping me awake.

What is going on? Why can't I have some peace! BEEP, BEEP. *WHAT is that noise! Why won't it stop? Just please stop. Leave me alone. Leave me alone in misery.* BEEP, BEEP. *I can't handle this anymore. Oh God, I can't handle this anymore. I just had surgery. I almost died!* BEEP, BEEP. *STOP! I can't do this* anymore! *I just can't! This is too much! I've had enough. I can't do this! I won't!* BEEP, BEEP. *AHHHHH!*

And come to find out—all those thoughts were not just thoughts anymore. Somewhere between my brain and my mouth, the medicines had connected the two so that I was saying everything I was thinking. My mother, exasperated and at her wits end, briskly walked out of the room. She went up to the nurses' desk and exclaimed, "You have to get in there! There's something really wrong with her!"

Promptly, four nurses rushed into the room to find me weeping. "What's wrong!" one of the nurses asked hurriedly.

"I can't do this anymore!" I screamed.

One nurse was at the beeping monster pushing buttons, one was patting my forehead, one was shuffling my covers around, and the other was holding my hand. I suddenly felt embarrassed. *Oh no, I'm being stupid. This isn't that big of a deal.* "I'm so sorry. I feel so stupid," I cried.

"Why? What do you mean?" a nurse worriedly asked.

"I'm making a big deal out of nothing. I'm fine. I'm so sorry. I feel so stupid." *Now I've gone and done it. Now everyone is worried about me. This is just so much. I didn't want to worry anyone.*

A nurse tried to comfort me, "Ohhh no, honey, you're doing much better than most people." After many repeats of me apologizing, "It's okays," pats of my legs, and rubbing of my forehead, I calmed down and finally passed out.

The next morning, barely daylight outside, my oncologist came in to check on me. Mom told him about the severe pain and my "episode," as she called it. He said the pain he could do something about, but the other part, he would have to refer me to someone with more expertise. He sent in another psychologist. I was so drugged I do not remember anything other than my mother and sister being upset because she had asked them to leave the room while we talked. I can only imagine what that lady heard that day. I was once again prescribed two more prescriptions. I did not care enough to ask what they were.

Later that day, my mother informed me of what was discovered with the surgery. My cancer had spread to two lymph nodes. Mom was very upset by that. At the time, I did not understand why. *What is a lymph node anyway? I don't care what a lymph node is. So what if a couple of lymph nodes have cancer? That doesn't surprise me. I have cancer. We already knew that. I don't understand what everyone is so shocked about.*

My stay in the hospital seemed to last forever. I did not want to eat, I did not want to talk, I did not want to watch TV. All I wanted to do was sleep. Three days later, I got tired of always sleeping and told Mom, "This sucks. I am always drowsy. I am ready to be back to normal." They took out my epidural and took me off my "button," which was a very lovely button that gave me morphine whenever I pushed it. They started me on oral medicines. The transition of taking me off intravenous pain medicine to giving me oral medicines resulted in the painkillers wearing off. Within an hour, I wanted my button back. They did not give it to me. I had to deal with oral medicines. That's what I asked for; that's what I got. Once I got the oral medicines, I was not as comfortable, but I was awake. I felt a little more like me.

The events and the aftermath of the surgery kept creeping into my mind. *When I woke up and heard someone tell me to calm down, I couldn't open my eyes. It was dark. I remember during my job shadowing of a hospital during high school, an anesthesiologist showed me how they tape the patient's eyes shut during sedation. Were mine taped shut? Then I felt someone pull something out of my throat, was that the actual breathing tube? Did I wake up during surgery? Then I blacked out. Then after that, why did that nurse have to tell me to breathe each breath? Does anesthesia not work on me? What happened?*

I was astonished at my first look at my new stomach when they changed my dressing later that afternoon. It was ugly. I had a vertical cut from the top of my pelvis to about four inches above my belly button. My stomach was lumpy and gruesome-looking.

My dad came to visit me during my stay. He seemed very upset and worried. He was there during my first attempt to get phlegm out of my chest. I couldn't cough, but I had fluid built up in my lungs. I could feel it. The nurse told me to sit up and exhale hard to try to get it up. It took about thirty minutes, but I finally got it. Then I passed out from exhaustion.

A few days into my stay, I was restless. I became tired of being there all together; I wanted to go home. They informed me of the tasks that I had to complete in order to go home. First was to take a shower. Thankfully, they had a seat to sit on, which I used the entire time. They tried to get me to eat; I refused.

With the next day came my next task. It was walking up and down the hallway. I made that my goal, striving as hard as I possibly could to accomplish that task. It was hard. I was ahead of their expected timeframe, but I wanted out of there. With every step, I had to push myself even harder, past the building pain, past the self-doubt. It took so long and so much effort to do something I could have done in a matter of seconds before, but I finally walked that hallway. After a long nap, they tried to get me to eat again. Once more, I refused.

That evening, I told Dr. Johnson that I had done all that he asked and was ready to go home. He smiled, stated he was proud of me, but then pointed out that I was missing one final step. I had not had a bowel movement because I had not eaten. My heart sank. I was going to have to eat. I hadn't eaten anything since my arrival. The idea of food, the idea of nourishment at such a time, was something I wanted to stay as far away from as possible. But now it was on my list to conquer in order to go home. So, I ate. I forced it down. I didn't eat much, but I ate nonetheless.

The next morning, I awoke to a surprise—a surprise that would normally not have been such a pleasant experience—however, I was thrilled to find that I had pooped myself. So thrilled that when Mom dropped my cellphone, I didn't even care. Before the pooping of the pants, I was quite insufferable and grouchy. The slipping of the phone would have brought on a fit of rage, but instead I was finally smiling for the first time since my arrival. I even joked, "You're lucky I just pooped." She didn't laugh. She didn't take it as a joke; she knew there was truth behind the comment. And she wasn't the happiest camper at that moment as I was trying to talk her into cleaning me up. I told her I didn't want the nurses to see me like that. They had already had to deal with me being so needy during my mental breakdown. I was already embarrassed enough from that whole ordeal. She insisted that's what they got paid to do. I told her I was embarrassed that I pooped the bed and didn't want them having to wipe my butt; I wanted her to do it. She gave a loud sigh and did what only a good mother would do. She wiped her grown child's butt. There is nothing quite like the love of a mother.

The entire time, I couldn't help but think I had conquered all of my obstacles. I was finally going home. I was being set free.

On July 25, my oncologist came in, gave me a kiss on my forehead, and said, "I'm so proud of you. You did it. You get to go home." *Finally.*

My people will live in safety, quietly at home. They will be at rest.
—Isaiah 32:18 NLT

12

Leiomyosarcoma

Throughout my stay in the hospital, I had finally started realizing that my life would change forever. Rather than going to my mom's and have someone take care of me while I recover, I decided I wanted to go to my apartment, my home. My mother was hesitant with my decision, but drove me to my apartment nonetheless. I wanted to be alone. I did not want someone caring about me when I could not care about myself.

I was to take it easy, stay in bed, and get plenty of rest. That is exactly what I did *not* do. My careless antics continued. I was up and about. I was driving. Not really caring to answer calls from my family. Not really caring to take care of myself at all.

The follow-up appointment with my oncologist was a week after my release. They removed my catheter, took out the staples on my incision, and then the doctor came in with the diagnosis. They finally had the results of what kind of cancer I had. *I will finally have some answers after all of this mess.*

He described the process of identifying cancer by drawing a house: a house with some tabs as "identifiers." He explained that they could not identify all the tabs or identifiers of my cancer. *Meaning what?*

Meaning my cancer is very rare in the fact that it cannot be fully identified. However, he did say that the best as they could identify, it was closest to leiomyosarcoma (lī-ō-mī-ō-sär-kō-mă) or LMS.

I was told that LMS is an aggressive, unpredictable, and reoccurring cancer. It is also an extremely rare cancer, especially in someone my age. *There we go again with rare. First it was rare that I have a fibroid at my age.* Well, I did. *Then it was even more rare that it is cancerous, especially at my age.* Well, it was. *And now my cancer is so rare that they can't even completely define it? What? That explains why the results from my first sample took so long. I haven't even gotten that back yet come to think of it.* I had a flashback of calling and screaming at the receptionist with the hospital that was testing my first sample during that horribly long "waiting game." I felt a tinge of guilt for taking it out on the poor lady.

My oncologist assured me that he had the best of the United States' sarcoma oncologists look at it, and they all agreed on the diagnosis and treatment plan. *But they don't exactly know what the diagnosis is! How are they going to treat this without even knowing for sure what it is? It obviously is not the leiomyo-whatever-it-is; it is just "close" to it. I don't understand what is happening. Why can't they tell what I have? They have never seen a cancer like this? Has no one had this cancer before? How is that even possible? They don't know what my cancer is. This is insane.*

There was a clinical trial that had recently started, and I had just missed the entry date, but my treatment was going to follow the same schedule. My doctor seemed happy about that. I was not. *A clinical trial? Trial? That sounds like they don't really know what they are doing if it is a trial. Do they not know how to fight this cancer? Am I going to be a guinea pig?*

Did I have any other option? No. I just had to trust that what was being done was the best possible care that I could receive at that time. That would have to be good enough. It was terrifying.

Treatment would consist of two different types of chemotherapy given weekly: Gemzar and Taxotere. It would be administered in cycles of three weeks. First week, Gemzar; second week, Gemzar and Taxotere. The third week would be a break from chemotherapy, but I would get a white blood cell booster shot, Neulasta, instead to help my immune system. Then start with the same cycle again. We would run this cycle six times. Eighteen weeks. Almost five months. That was the plan. America's best sarcoma oncologists had all agreed on it.

My oncologist stressed the point that chemotherapy is extremely hard on a person. He explained that the point of chemotherapy was to kill the cancer cells, but there was a catch. It kills the good cells along with the bad cells. He also explained that when a patient gets chemotherapy intravenously (through your vein), it runs the risk of collapsing the vein after repeated exposure to chemotherapy. In order to save my veins, I had to get a port, which was a catheter under my skin on my chest.

He explained that the cancer treatment consisted of more than just surgery and chemotherapy. It would encompass my whole body and mind. Cancer patients do best when they stay positive. Their head game has a lot to do with how well they respond to treatment. *How can anyone stay positive during this? How is that possible?* They gave me a huge red binder with tons of information about chemotherapy: side effects, what to eat, what not to eat, what to expect, when to contact your doctor, just tons of information. I barely looked at it; it was too overwhelming.

The appointment to get my port placed into my chest was in a week. Chemotherapy would start a week after that. *So fast. All happening so fast. I just had a hysterectomy. And now a port and then chemo? Too fast!*

I asked if I would lose my hair.

They responded with an adamant *yes*. It was said with such certainty that I was taken back. I felt as though I had just been slapped across the face. *Wait. What? I'm going to lose my hair? Surely not…this can't be…*

As I sat in shock, the conversation carried on. Since I had a full hysterectomy, my ovaries were removed, along with everything else. That meant no estrogen. My oncologist explained that they were still unsure if my cancer was estrogen-fed; therefore, he did not want to prescribe me estrogen. He warned me that my body was going to enter a harsh menopause. He explained that my symptoms would be worse than normal menopause due to my body being suddenly forced into it at such a young age.

My body did not have a chance to get used to gradually losing the estrogen; it lost all of it with a slice of the knife during surgery.

He made it pretty clear that it was going to be miserable.

My first hot flash was at Olive Garden after the checkup. I was sitting at the table with my Mom when I suddenly felt...weird.

"Oh no," I said as I sat down my fork.

"What?" Mom looked at me, confused.

I sat and stared at my cheesecake. The room was spinning. I suddenly felt extremely light-headed. I felt as though I was going to throw up, turn inside out, and faint all at the same time. "I feel weird. Something's wrong," I whispered.

"What is it?" She was looking worried at this point.

"I don't know...something's happening," I said between panting breathes.

Loudly, she asked, "Well, what is it!"

"Just give me a minute. I don't know. Something's happening." There was a slow build of heat from deep within me. "Is it hot in here?" I asked.

"No, it's not. Are you okay?"

The heat had spread throughout my entire torso. "It's hot in here." I started fanning the neck of my shirt.

She handed me a glass of water and said, "You're really red."

By this point, my insides were boiling. I wanted to dump the water on my chest. I wanted to take all my clothes off. I wanted to lie down on the cold tile floor. The heat was so overwhelming I felt I couldn't breathe. I grabbed my napkin and started waving it in my face, breathing harder and faster.

"You're having a hot flash," Mom stated.

"I am?" I asked in confusion.

"That's what it looks like to me," she replied.

Slowly the heat started to fade away, and I began to feel myself again.

That was a hot flash? That was flipping horrible. I better not have to deal with those very often. He said I would have them a lot, and they would be bad—but dang, I wasn't expecting that.

As we finished our meal, I couldn't help but think about the possibility of me losing my hair. It loomed over me, as if a dark cloud. *I'm going to lose my hair. No ifs or maybes. She said it like it was a for-sure thing. That sure doesn't help me "stay positive," as they said I was supposed to. Am I going to look like one of those dead skeletons walking around in the waiting room? Is that going to happen to me? How can that be? Me. This is happening to me. Me. My hair. My life. Me.*

A couple of weeks later, I finally decided to see what I was up against. I found some resources on leiomyosarcoma. It is a type of soft-tissue sarcoma. Soft-tissue sarcoma is a cancer of the connective tissues, such as muscles, tendons, nerves, fat, and blood vessels. Sarcoma in itself is rare, with only a few thousand cases a year in the US. Leiomyosarcoma is an extremely rare cancer, making up less than 1 percent of the total sarcoma diagnoses. Most oncologists never see leiomyosarcoma throughout their entire career.

Come to find out, it is so rare that there has not been enough research on how to cure it. With what little research they do have, they found it to be a "resistant cancer"; meaning, it does not typically respond to chemotherapy or radiation. Due to the fact that the cancer is typically unresponsive, the best option is surgery, with chemotherapy as a backup. *What's the point if it doesn't work?*

I also discovered that it is one of the most aggressive cancers and is extremely unpredictable. My cancer was high grade, also known as poorly differentiated. That means the cells were very abnormal, with no resemblance to any tissue in the body—which, in turn, means it's dangerous and very unpredictable.

The recurrence rate is high; meaning, it is likely to come back, especially if it had spread to lymph nodes. Mine had. My cancer was stage IV, the most advanced stage. When a cancer gets to the lymph system, it spreads much quicker and easier to other parts of the body. There is no cure for stage IV leiomyosarcoma. It was mostly likely to metastasize in the lungs, other organs, or limbs. But it could show up anywhere. Anywhere in the body, any soft tissue.

It normally hits women who are fifty or sixty years old, and the survival rate is among the lowest of all sarcomas. The statistics read that 14 percent of people survive five years after diagnosis. One case study I looked at had sixteen people that were diagnosed, and 93 percent of them died. I did the math: 14.88 people died. That's close enough to say that fifteen people died. One person survived five years. One. The bomb hit.

I was so stricken with fear that I was afraid to discuss it with anyone. I finally got the courage to mention it to Mom and learned a few more things. Unbeknownst to me, my mother had bluntly asked my oncologist team, "Is it going to kill her?"

One of my cancer team members stated, "Yes, but not this time." Mom said that she had already looked up the statistics and anticipated the answer but wanted to hear it from the medical team.

In my spiral downward, I finally had something to grasp and hang on to. Fear. Submerging and suffocating fear. *Six in one million people are diagnosed with leiomyosarcoma; 14 percent live five years. Most die. How can all of these statistics be the worst of the worse? This seems all so unreal. I'm so young. I haven't accomplished anything yet. How can this be? I'm going to die.*

Resources

"Leiomyosarcoma," last updated July 2011, http://leiomyosarcoma.info/.

"Sarcoma Information for Leiomyosarcoma Families," last updated August 2017, http://www.leiomyosarcoma.org/soft-tissue-leiomyosarcoma/.

> *But Jesus looked at them and said, "With man this is impossible, but with God all things are possible."*
> —Matthew 19:26 ESV

13

More Antics

Only a few weeks after my surgery, I went out drinking and dancing. The next morning, I woke up in another town. The crowd I was with had obviously found a new place to crash. As I stumbled around trying to find a bathroom, I noticed my incision was sore, and it felt *different*. When I found the bathroom, I raised my shirt to see the damage. Several of my stitches were busted open. As I slid my hand over my newly deformed incision, I had a flashback of me dancing on the dance floor with a drink in my hand. I had felt a popping sensation on my stomach. At the time, I had thought, *Was that a stitch?* I slammed my drink and headed toward the bar for another.

I looked at myself in the mirror. *That looks like me, but she doesn't feel like me. Who is "me" anymore? I don't know who I am anymore. I don't want to be "me" anymore. That "me" went out the window. There is no "me."* I felt completely disconnected to everything I had ever known. My life was no longer the same happy, levelheaded, good-choice, good-girl life I had once lived. I was now standing in a complete stranger's dirty bathroom, with people I really barely even knew, still drunk from the night before.

Prior to my diagnosis, I was one of the most responsible and dependable people I knew. I was valedictorian of my graduating high school class, I graduated college with honors, I always tried hard to do the right thing. *What has happened to me?*

Everything I knew to be true and stable had been ripped away from me. I felt as though my life was no longer mine. It was cancer's.

I did not know who I was anymore. I lost my character. I lost my values. I felt as though I was losing every aspect of my life—of me.

*For the Son of Man has come to seek
and to save that which was lost.*
—Luke 19:10 AMP

14

Down Here with You

I had been taking classes for months in order to get an Early Childhood certificate, known as a CDA. I had already received my bachelor's degree in elementary education, but had been motivated to further my education for work. All the classes and assignments were complete; there was just one last step to complete the process. An administrator would meet with me to give a written exam and an interview. I was to wait on the call to schedule the appointment, and then the certification would be complete.

One day at work, I received a phone call from a friendly lady reminding me of my appointment at noon at the local library. *What?*

She stated that she had called my cell phone several weeks earlier and spoke with my mother to schedule a time and place. She said my mother had taken the message and said she would get it to me. *Uh-oh. Wait, when would Mom answer my phone? Oh, it must have been during my hysterectomy.*

The lady on the phone asked if I was still able to make the appointment. Considering she was from out of state and already meeting another girl for the same assessment, I agreed, not putting too much care into it. *If I pass, I pass. If I fail, I fail. What does it matter now anyway?*

I gave my mother a quick call to see if she remembered what this lady was talking about. Mom said, "Well, yes, I told you about it and put it in your purse while we were at the hospital. Don't you remember?" I was a little annoyed that Mom had expected me to remember considering the medications I was on, but the appointment was that day at noon, and that was that.

At noon, I made my way down to the local library, found the front desk to ask where I should go, and was directed into a small room in the back of the library. There I found an older lady and a woman about the same age as me.

My mind was reeling with my life's circumstances, and I found it difficult to concentrate, but I completed the test, not really knowing if I had blown it or if I had managed to muddle my way through. It was then time for the interview. I opted to go first, so the younger woman stepped out of the room. The older lady asked me several questions, which I surprisingly managed to have answers for.

After the interview, she started talking about her personal life. She said that when she was younger, she had an overwhelming feeling that she was supposed to go overseas. She was not sure why she felt that strong urge, but she felt that God was telling her to, so away she went. It was there that she did some works for God and then returned to the States. I found it odd that she was randomly telling me this story, but I sat and listened.

I didn't quite understand what her point was until she made it clear that she was led there for a reason. Sadly, I cannot remember what the reason was; however, she made it clear that it was very significant. She explained that God has a plan for everything and that everything has a purpose.

Soon after that story, she began talking to me about how my experience is happening for a reason. She spoke as though she knew more than I had told her. *Did Mom tell her what was going on when she took that message? Even if she did tell her, this lady is not only talking to me as though she knows my circumstances. She is speaking like she knows me—I mean really knows me.*

She told me something that surprised me, something that I had never even considered before. She said, "You are going to be fine. Your story is going to inspire so many people."

My story? I'm going to have a story? I don't even know if I'm going to make it through this, let alone help other people. That does sound kind of nice, though, but I doubt it. What is happening here? Is this for real?

How does she know all of this? Why does it feel different? I'm not even really sure if I believe in God, yet I'm getting a strange sense of a higher power here. Is this from God? Is God talking through this lady? What is happening?

Next thing I knew, she had me up out of my chair, and she was hugging me. It was not a quick I'm-glad-I got-to-meet-you kind of hug. It was a long hug that felt warm and comforting. She started crying. "I'm so sorry this is happening to you." I had heard that enough that it could have seemed like a normal statement, although I had not had anyone tell me that while they were crying and holding me. While standing there in her embrace, I thought, *She feels like my Aunt Gayle.*

My Aunt Gayle had died in a car wreck years earlier. We had been very close. I had a flashback of my joyful anticipation of my Aunt Gayle's routine goodbyes as a child. First was a big bear hug, much like the one I was in at the very moment. Next was the Eskimo kisses, where we would rub our cheeks together in a circular motion. Finally, we would end with giggles while giving butterfly kisses, where we would bat our eyelashes while trying to tilt our heads in a way that allowed our eyelashes to touch.

I was brought back to reality when I heard the lady say, "Everything happens for a reason. It's going to be okay. You're going to be okay." It was so odd that I was getting a sense of comfort from a statement by a complete stranger.

How does this lady know that I'm going to be okay? And why do I believe her?

Then she said something that made my breath get caught in my throat. "I wish I could be down here with you."

Did I just hear her right? Down here with you? Down from where? What state was she from? Why would she want to be here with me if she doesn't know me? Down from where? Why do I keep getting this feeling that she knows me? I've never met this lady before in my life, yet I feel like I know her.

She stopped hugging me and explained that after her hysterectomy, she had vacuumed, and it had caused her some complications with her healing. She insisted for me not to vacuum for several weeks.

She told me to get someone else to do my vacuuming for me while I recovered. *What a random statement—not to vacuum? Who is this lady!*

I responded with a simple, "Okay." *Is this lady crazy?*

She embraced me again and began to cry this time, saying, "I love you."

Oddly, with hearing her say those words, I felt it. I felt an overwhelming sense of comfort in her arms. I felt it was something more than a stranger hugging me. I felt it was more than some batty old lady acting crazy. It was more. There was more in that room. There was more to this situation. I can't explain it, and it may sound crazy, but I just knew. I could feel it.

I left the room in a daze. While on the walk to my car, I was contemplating whether to tell anyone. Would they think I'm crazy? Would they believe me? Would they think that it's all in my head? *Is it all in my head? That lady told me she loved me. Like she really knew me. Who tells a complete stranger that they love them while hugging and crying? She wasn't a stranger, was she? And then she said "down here with you." Down here. Down here from somewhere "up there." But from where? Heaven?*

When I got to my car, I sat in the driver's seat and called my mom. "I just had a really weird experience." My voice sounded confused.

Mom hesitantly said, "Okaaaaay?"

"This lady who gave me the test acted like she really knew me. I mean *really* knew me." I wanted to tell her all the details but felt it would sound less real, less meaningful if I said them out loud. I wanted to hang on to the feeling of comfort that I had oddly gotten from this peculiar circumstance.

Mom sat silent, waiting.

"Mom, I think I just met an angel, and I think it might have been Aunt Gayle." A fearful thought crossed my mind, *Am I so desperate for comfort that I really believe my Aunt Gayle would really make a trip from heaven to visit me through a stranger?*

Instead of responding with what I had expected, Mom simply said, "If Gayle could have found a way to get down here to you, she would. You were her very favorite, and she just loved you so much. She would do anything to get down here to you."

I got goose bumps. *Mom just said "down here"—twice. Is that a sign?*

I had a sense of comfort that I had found nowhere else, and it was from the most unlikely source, a complete stranger. Was this really a heavenly intervention? Or was it simply some batty old lady trying her best to touch the life of a lost soul? No matter what it was, I decided I was going to hold on to what I felt—a sense of comfort, a sense of purpose, a sense of a future.

> *"For I know the plans I have for you," says the Lord. "They are plans for good and not for disaster, to give you a future and a hope."*
> —Jeremiah 29:11 NLT

15

Port Placement

"What the *heck*, Jessi! You're almost two hours late!" Mom yelled as she rushed out her front door to meet me in her driveway. And she was cursing.

I quickly responded lightheartedly and maybe a little too loudly, "Oh well, Mom, it's not like they can start without me!" I began laughing as I stumbled out of the driver seat of my car. It was time for my port placement—well, technically, past time.

"Are you *drunk*!" Her eyes were on fire. She was furious.

"I don't know," was all I could think to say.

After realizing I had driven the thirty-minute drive to her house, she exclaimed, "And you *drove*?"

I shrugged.

"It's like you just don't give a crap about anything!"

Yes, I thought. *That is correct. I, in fact, do* not *care—about anything.* I heard the desperation in her voice, which was the reason I kept my thoughts to myself as she got into the driver's seat, and we started the two-hour drive.

"You *reek* of liquor, Jessi. What did you drink?" she asked in disgust.

I had some blurred memories of several mixed drinks and more than a few shots of hard liquors. "Oh…just some stuff. I don't really remember," I replied honestly.

"Who were you with? Did they know you were having surgery today?"

Thinking back on the night before, I remember that I had actually confided in one person that I had been diagnosed with cancer. I had decided not to give details. The word *cancer* was enough. "Yeah, I told them," I answered.

She was still heated. "And they did this? The night before your surgery? What kind of friends are these? They could have at least made sure you got up on time." I had a flashback of me attempting to set my alarm before passing out. It obviously didn't work.

I shrugged. Mom's phone started ringing. It was my sister, Laveda Dawn. "Are you close?" Laveda asked.

Mom exclaimed, "No! We're just *now* leaving!"

Dawn hesitantly asked, "Is she singing?"

"Yes, she's singing," Mom replied, irritated.

"Wow, well, she's in quite a good mood today," Dawn replied.

"She's *drunk*!" Mom shot me a look that could kill.

Dawn questioned, "She's drunk?" as if she was expecting a punch line to a joke.

"*Yes*! She showed up an hour and a half late—drunk!" Mom's face was red.

Dawn gave a quiet, "Oh, no."

They got off the phone. I tried to make light of the situation by making jokes and laughing. It was the first time that the two-hour drive to the oncologist wasn't silent.

When we pulled into the parking garage, Dawn was standing outside of her vehicle, waiting. As I got out of the car, I stumbled and couldn't help but giggle. Dawn was suddenly there, helping me up. She put her arm around me to help me walk and smiled at me. I'm not sure if she was smiling because we had finally arrived or if she was relieved to see a smile on my face for the first time in a very long time.

"What have you done *now*, dear sister?" she asked as she helped me walk out of the parking garage.

"Oh, you know. Mom is mad at me."

Laveda lightly said, "Yeah she sure is. You're lucky you made it here in one piece." After realizing she was right, I started laughing. Dawn joined in on the laughter. When I turned around to see if

Mom was in earshot, I could have sworn I caught a glance of a smile on her face.

By the time we got into the correct room, I was walking by myself. I signed in and entered the prep room after a short wait. The realization of what was about to happen was sobering me quite quickly.

Up until that point, I had done my very best to avoid all emotions when it came to one of the scariest truths. I was going to be a chemotherapy patient, and today was the day I would get the port for it. That reality must have brought back a wisp of the real me because I suddenly became embarrassed that I was such a mess. My family knew it, but I felt secure enough with them that I trusted they would not judge. What if the hospital staff could tell I was intoxicated? I did not want strangers judging my decisions.

"Do you think they will be able to tell?" I worriedly asked.

"Well, yes, they will be able to tell! You reek of whiskey!" Mom loudly exclaimed. I glanced around the prep room to see if anyone had heard my mother loudly rat me out.

"Shhhh! I don't want them to know I'm drunk," I worried out loud.

A nurse came up to start an IV. She leaned in close as another nurse was asking the routine list of questions. *Dang it, they are going to smell it on my breath.* I tried to answer while looking away from the nurses but soon realized that appeared very awkward and odd. I then answered a couple of questions covering my mouth. I got a couple of odd glances for that technique, so I resorted to answering as fast and short as I could. I was pretty positive they could smell it on me, despite my best attempts, but no one said anything.

The surgery was supposed to be a quick, painless, an in-and-out procedure. They would give local anesthetics and conscious sedation. Meaning, they would numb the area and give me some sedatives to make me sleepy and not remember the procedure. Well, unfortunately, I did realize what was going on, and I remember every part.

I felt and vividly remember the scalpel cutting into my flesh. After I cried out in pain, they gave me more sedatives. After the extra dose, I then remember the doctor and nurse chatting about the doctor's daughter's birthday party the weekend before.

Next thing I knew, the doctor was painfully shoving the tube down under my skin through a hole on my upper right chest. I remember the doctor having problems getting it where it needed to be, so he did what any other doctor would do: he shoved harder. It hurt. The anesthesiologist kept asking if I was okay.

There was a television showing a picture of his progress. When I tried to turn my head to see the TV to figure out if he was almost done, he would tell me to turn my head back the other way. I started wishing I had been more drunk; maybe that would have helped numb it.

Then, finally, it was done.

A male nurse wheeled me out to the recovery room and brought in my mom and sister. While I transferred myself from the gurney to the hospital bed, the nurse told them, "She's had enough sedatives that a normal person would be in a coma."

I told them, "It didn't work. I knew what they were doing the entire time."

The nurse nervously said, "She may say she remembers everything, but she doesn't."

I gave him a nasty look. *Oh, really? I don't remember? What a jerk. He doesn't know what I do or do not remember.*

Within minutes, I was walking around the room, ready to be released, but they insisted per hospital protocol that I had to be wheeled out in a wheelchair. I was mad that I had to endure the pain and listen to the conversation about the doctor's daughter's birthday party while they were unaware that I was quite aware. I was even more upset that the nurse had discredited me and claimed that I did not remember what I had. Then to act like I wasn't capable of walking out of the hospital when I was clearly walking fine around the room made me even more irritated.

As they wheeled me out of the hospital, I couldn't help but wonder, *Why do I have such a high tolerance for pain medicines? Was it because I was still intoxicated? No, that couldn't be it because I woke up during the hysterectomy, and I was completely sober. Was it because I've been drinking so much lately? Does that do that?* I had no idea that I would finally have an answer years later when my dentist warned that Ambien, a sleep aid, causes problems with anesthesia during surgeries. It was at that moment I finally put it together. I had been taking it for years before cancer.

That sucks.

> *Look, today I am giving you the choice*
> *between a blessing and a curse!*
> —Deuteronomy 11:26 NLT

16

Plunging Headfirst

After my port placement, I had a week before starting chemotherapy. I was to rest and let my body heal as much as it could while it had the chance. Chemotherapy would hinder the healing process, and there was a lot to heal, considering I just had the hysterectomy a matter of weeks ago. I knew I should stop my dumb antics, but that's not exactly what happened.

During that crucial week, I was no longer sliding downhill. I had plunged headfirst, crashing downward wild and fast. I'm going to be honest and tell you what I would prefer not to.

I was given several rules from my oncologist to ensure I would heal as best as I could before injecting a poison into my body. I followed none of them. I was told I was to rest and let my body recoup. Rule avoided. I was told how to take careful precautions with my bandages to avoid infection. Rule forgotten. I was told not to drink alcohol while consuming the painkillers. Rule broken. I was in the deepest despair of my life without even acknowledging it.

Just a couple of months earlier, I had felt I had complete control over my life. I thought I had it all together. Suddenly two months later, I was a week away from starting the scariest and most horrifying experience of my life. Chemotherapy was a whole realm of horror that I couldn't bring myself to face. I had, along with most of society, a preexisting perception of chemotherapy. Chemotherapy was a long, drawn-out, tortuous ordeal that ended in death.

I had no idea what my feelings were at the time because I did not allow myself to feel. But the relentless thoughts kept coming:

Am I going to die? Am I going to be dead a month from now? Will chemotherapy kill me? Will the cancer kill me? As soon as these thoughts would enter my mind, I would try to push down the feelings that accompanied them. I felt they would overwhelm and overcome me. They would take hold and pull me down so deep I wouldn't be able to breathe. They would suffocate me.

Seeing and hearing my family's fears brought up fears of my own. They were scared I was going to die. No matter how hard they forced themselves to say, "You're going to be okay," I knew they were lying. They were just as scared as I was. When I had to talk to my loved ones, I was short and rude, pushing them away. All they wanted was to be with me or even hear from me, yet I avoided them. Just hearing their voices brought feelings that were too real. Seeing how worried they were brought feelings of guilt. It was my fault they were worried. It was all because of me, my cancer.

For His strength is made perfect in our weakness.
—2 Corinthians 12:9

17

Chemotherapy

On the morning of the first chemotherapy day, August 12, 2011, I woke up in my apartment early, before my alarm. I felt as though I was almost having an out-of-body experience as I went through the mundane routine of getting ready for the day—disconnected, numb, shocked, worried.

As I brushed my hair, I couldn't help but wonder if this was the last time, I was going to be able to brush my hair. *Will it fall out today?* I gave my cat a kiss goodbye and headed out the door.

The thirty-minute drive to my Mom's house was shorter than normal. My mind was lost in thoughts. *The day is here. Already here. Chemo day. This is it.* I kept trying to push down the feelings, the worries, in an attempt to desperately remain in my numb state that I had grown familiar with, but it was harder this time.

When I arrived at Mom's, she was busy getting ready. I wasn't late this time, although I wish I would have been. I didn't want to go at all, let alone on time. Mom drove the two-hour drive to the cancer center. She tried to make small talk; I wasn't participating. More feelings and worries came creeping up, gnawing at me. *Just keep it together. Don't break down now. You can't.*

When we arrived at the cancer center, we met Dawn in the parking lot. After a quick hello, we headed inside. We went to a new floor, the "chemo floor." That, in itself, was rather intimidating. A whole floor of the building was dedicated to this scary event. When we walked into the new waiting room, there was the usual crowd of ill-looking people. The difference this time: more of them were bald.

That bothered me. I did not want to lose my hair. *Why do I have to do this? I don't want to do this. Stop, just get through this.*

After what seemed a short minute, a nurse called my name, and we were guided into another set of hallways. They were not the normal set of hallways. These hallways were between what I would describe as cubicles. The cubicle walls were a little taller than a normal office cubicle, but they did not go up to the ceiling. They were small and close together. It gave the area a sense of openness, yet the cubicle doors were closed which provided privacy. *Good, we will be alone.*

While walking back, the nurse asked me for my name and birth date. *Uhhhh, my birth date? Why am I drawing a blank?* My mind seemed cloudy. "Jessica Bell, June 29, 1986." *Right? What happens if I answer wrong?*

It must have been correct because she continued to lead us back to a cubicle. As I walked into the small room, I froze while looking at its contents. *This is the chemotherapy room. This is where it will happen.*

The room was small. There was a large brown reclining chair with two regular smaller chairs to either side. There was a TV on top of a set of cabinets and a sink in the corner. It surprisingly looked like a somewhat comfortable space. I, however, was not comfortable at all. I was not comfortable with being there regardless of how it appeared. I was actually on the opposite side of the spectrum. This was the last place on earth I wanted to be.

Mom and Dawn both took one of the side chairs as I stood and stared at what was obviously my chair. The brown reclining chair was the "chemo chair." That spot wasn't for my mom; it wasn't for my sister. It was mine. *That spot is for me. That chemo chair is meant for me. Me alone.*

With that realization while staring at the chair, an overwhelming amount of feelings suddenly came barging through my wall of indifference and made itself quite known. There was a deep pressure pushing itself up, catching in my throat. I couldn't stop it. *Keep calm. Don't freak out.* My head started spinning. *I'm getting chemotherapy.*

My chest became tight. *Me. It's happening to me.* I sat down in the chair in an attempt to regain myself. *Just breathe.*

Mom and Dawn were getting themselves settled. *Keep it together. Don't do it. Keep it together.* I was trying to settle myself too, but it wasn't working. I was horrified. The first feeling I think I had admitted to myself experiencing, and it was only because I was forced to feel it. It was not that I "let myself" feel it. The overwhelming fear was there, and it was loud. *I don't want to do this. I shouldn't have to be here. I'm going to die. I have cancer. Why do I feel so weird? There's a pressure, a strong pressure...in my throat.*

All the feelings I had never allowed myself to feel were right there—in my throat. Right there, ready to explode. I felt as though I was holding in an enormous amount of pressure, and one little drip would make the entire dam break, releasing an overwhelming flood of emotions. I was close to breaking. One little drip, and all control would be lost. *Don't think about it, don't think about it...cancer...no, don't think about it... I'm getting chemotherapy. Don't do this.* My control was slipping. I became even more scared, realizing that I could no longer suppress the feelings.

Suddenly a couple of older ladies pushing a cart came to our door and asked if we would like any refreshments. My mother and sister were pleased to get a cup of coffee. I, however, was lost in my inner state of turmoil. The two ladies were on their way to the next cubicle when I looked down and realized that I was somehow now holding a juice.

My mind was reeling. *Will the chemotherapy be a nasty concoction like a witch's brew? How long is it going to take? Don't think about it. I don't want to be here. My chest is hurting. Will the chemotherapy hurt? Chemotherapy...chemotherapy. I'm getting chemotherapy. Today. Don't think about it! It's happening now. The time is here. Why is my chest hurting so bad?*

I could no longer simply push the feelings down. There was no more room; they were boiling over. I was suddenly being forced to confront reality. *I'm going to be a chemotherapy patient. I have cancer. I'm going to die. My chest hurts bad.*

I could no longer deny it. Something was wrong. My chest had really started to hurt. *Why is my chest hurting? Is there something wrong with my port? They said the tube of my port is running to my heart. Oh my gosh, what if it has slipped and is poking my heart? Oh no. That's what's wrong. My port is poking my heart. This could be serious. No, just calm down.*

I sat and stared at Mom and Dawn while they were having small talk, oblivious to the hell I was enduring. They were so close to me, yet I felt as though I was light-years away from them. Alone.

Ouch. It really is hurting now. It's getting hard to breathe. I need to tell someone. No, you're overreacting. Everything's fine. But what if it's not fine? Ugh, it really hurts. What if my port really is poking my heart? TELL SOMEONE.

Without realizing, I had suddenly blurted out, "My chest hurts." Mom and Dawn stopped talking midconversation and looked at me, wide-eyed. *Why are they looking at me like that? It really is bad, isn't it? I knew it! Something's seriously wrong!*

Mom asked "Where is it hurting at?"

My mind was racing. *Chemotherapy…poison…me…*

"My heart. My heart is hurting. I can't breathe," I quickly rambled. *Will my hair fall out within minutes? Hours? Days? I'm going to lose my hair. You're not going to lose your hair! I'm going to die!*

Mom and Dawn were sitting there calmly watching me. *You're just sitting there fine while I am the one going through hell! You have no idea! You're not dealing with this! I am!*

"Do you want me to get the nurse?" Laveda worriedly asked.

I wanted to scream, *No, I don't want you to get a nurse!* But instead, "I don't know…maybe," came out in a panicked voice. "I feel dizzy and nauseous. I can't breathe. My heart is really hurting." *I'm going to lose my hair. I'm going to look like one of those walking skeletons. I hear someone crying. I want to cry. Don't cry. Don't cry.* DON'T CRY.

"Jessi, you're having a panic attack," Mom calmly stated.

I looked at Mom. She was so calm. "A what!" I asked doubtfully. The thoughts that were quickly racing through my mind were random and offbeat. *A panic attack? What in the world is she talking about? No, it is not a panic attack. My port is poking my heart. I have to have chemotherapy. I have cancer. It's not a panic attack. That's dumb.*

Of my prior twenty-five years, I had never experienced a panic attack. I had always thought it was just "in someone's head," a result of their own doing. Avoidable. Overrated. Not a big deal.

Mom repeated, "A panic attack." She turned to Laveda and said matter-of-factly. "Gayle used to have them."

IT'S NOT A PANIC ATTACK! Oh my gosh, my chest hurts bad. I'm going to die. I'm having a heart attack. The tube is poking my heart. Something is seriously wrong.

Mom and Dawn then began a conversation about how horrible panic attacks were and started to share their own experiences with panic attacks. Their conversation annoyed me. *It is not a panic attack! I don't have panic attacks. This is SERIOUS!* In the midst of their conversation, I loudly snapped, "How do you know my port isn't poking my heart!"

After that question, they promptly stopped talking, shot a quick glance at each other out the side of their eyes, and silently exchanged that "yeah, she's having a panic attack" look. They slowly turned their heads toward me, eyes wide.

I know what you're thinking! You don't believe me. But this is serious!

Mom comfortingly said, "Jessi, your port's not poking your heart. You said he could see what he was doing on the TV screen. He would have made sure that it was in its right place."

I sat there quiet for a second. *She's right. He did see it on the TV.* My mind racing, I blurted, "Yeah, okay. But how do you know the tube that goes to my heart hasn't moved and is *now* poking my heart?" I exclaimed.

They don't believe me. No one ever believes me. And look, I have cancer. No one believes me when I tell them something is wrong. In an attempt to help them understand the severity of the issue, I said, "My heart is *really* hurting."

They were both quiet for a moment, each quickly assessing the situation. Sure, it was possible that the port had become dislodged and was causing problems, but not likely. They were both trying to find that one thing to say to calm me down.

Mom had it. "Jessi, if it was a possibility of it poking your heart, don't you think that they would have scanned you and checked that it was okay?"

Laveda, who was obviously reassured herself with Mom's reasonable answer, quickly chimed in, "Yes, Jessi. She's right. They would have checked if it was a possibility."

Okay, maybe she's right. "Then why is my chest hurting so bad? Am I having a heart attack?"

Before someone could respond, a new nurse came in, introduced herself, and explained that she would be getting me "set up." *Set up? It's happening. It's happening now. Oh God, it's happening.* She asked how I was feeling.

"I don't know..." *I don't want to make a big deal of this. But something isn't right. What if she doesn't believe me? Doctors don't have the best reputation for believing my symptoms are serious. I'm not going to say anything. I'm going to keep this to myself.*

Mom decided to take control. "Well, she's not doing good."

The nurse looked at me. "Oh no, what's going on?"

I glanced over at Mom, who had just ratted me out. *I don't want to tell anyone. What if it is a panic attack? I'll feel dumb. This hurts bad, though. I can't, though. I can't admit anything is wrong.* The feelings were more forceful than ever. They were right there, making me teeter on the edge. I was about to lose it. *I can't do this.*

Impatient, Mom forcefully prodded, "Tell her, Jessi!"

I quickly rattled off, "I can't breathe. My head is spinning, and my chest is hurting. I feel like I ran a mile." That was it. The dam broke. That was the last drip. Admitting I was not fine was more than I could bear. All the feelings I had held down for so long suddenly came busting through, boiling upward. They were loose. They were uncontrollable. I started to cry. *I can't stop it. It's too much.* Tears streaming down my face, I looked up at the nurse.

"This can be pretty traumatic. A lot of people are nervous when they get their first chemo treatment, but it will get better." She patted my hand.

I continued to cry. Fear, worry, anxiety, sadness, anger, denial—they were all suddenly there. There were there and strong. I wasn't able to control them anymore. It was too much. *I'm too young for this. I'm going to die a young woman. I haven't even done anything with my life. My family is going to be sad. I don't want to be here. I hate this. I don't want this. I don't want cancer. This isn't my fault. This is unfair. I don't want chemotherapy. No one understands what I'm going through. I can't do this. I can't handle this. This is too much for me. I'm done. I can't. Just can't do this. No more. I just can't. I'm going to die.*

Mom explained, "She hasn't been acknowledging anything that has been happening, and I think it's finally starting to hit her." As the nurse watched me sob uncontrollably, she agreed that's probably what the problem was.

Hearing the nurse agree I was having a panic attack made me feel a bit better. *Okay, maybe that's it then. But do panic attacks really cause this much pain? Is this really all in my head?*

"Let me get a hold of the doctor and see if we can't get you something to make you feel better," the nurse calmly said before walking out.

Whew. She believes me. That's a relief. This place is different. They actually believe me.

Before too long, the nurse was back with a little pill that would "help me feel better." Within fifteen minutes, I felt immensely better. I was still worried, but my pain had subsided. I had gained control of my feelings again and managed to stop crying. I felt a little better after letting some of the pressure out, and now it was time to deal with the situation. *No more crying. You're going to get chemotherapy. Keep it together now. It's time to be strong.*

Next thing I knew, Susan, my doctor's right hand, was at the door, checking on me. Seeing her concern made me feel a sense of embarrassment. *I'm fine. And here I have caused more people to worry about me.* Less than an hour after Susan left, but sooner than I had wanted, the nurse was there ready to begin the dreaded process. *It's time.*

She opened at least ten different packages, making sure not to contaminate anything, carefully placing each in its thought-out spot on the roll caddy: gloves, needles, tubes, gauze pads, and an assortment of unknown pieces.

She opened a long plastic tube with a flat circle on the end, did something to make a popping noise, and moved my shirt to look at my port. You could visibly see a large bump under my skin, under my scar. She began rubbing the flat part of the stick onto my chest. "This is to sterilize the area," she responded to my questioning look. It smelled of rubbing alcohol. She kept rubbing. *Okay, it has to be clean by now, lady.* She must have rubbed the tube on my chest for a good twenty seconds. After she was finally done with the sterilizing stick, she quickly twisted some tubes together, connected a needle, and asked me to lie back and relax.

Relax!

I heard her, "One...two...three." On three, I felt the needle enter my skin. *That wasn't so bad*, I thought. She wasn't done. She pulled outward on the needle just a hair, still leaving the needle under my skin, wiggled it around, and pushed inward. She did this a couple of times until she said, "Okay." *Okay, good, she must have got it.* She explained that there is a dime-sized cushion part in the center of the port that the needle has to hit. With the port just being placed a week ago, the tissue above the port was still swollen and hard to feel exactly where the needle should go, but she said she got it.

She then peeled the back off of what looked like a very large clear sticker and covered almost my entire chest with it. She stuck a syringe into the end of the tube that was connected to the needle in my chest. "This is to flush your port. You will taste this as I inject it. Some people say they despise the taste while others say it tastes like citrus." She started to inject the fluid, and I noticed a powerful burning at my port. No taste, just burning.

"How does that feel?" she asked.

I didn't say anything for a moment. I was contemplating whether to mention that it was painful or to just deal with it. I had already caused enough problems that I didn't want to complain anymore. *If this is part of it, it's got to be done.* The burning suddenly got worse.

She stood looking at me, waiting for me to answer her question.

"It hurts, but I think I can handle it," I replied.

She immediately stopped injecting the fluid and stated, "Hmm, it shouldn't hurt at all."

Great, what now?

She took off the large sticker, pulled out the needle, and left the room for a while, saying she needed more supplies. When she returned, she went through the whole process of opening the numerous packages and getting everything sat in its appointed place once again. She popped another one of those sterilizing sticks and cleaned my chest again for another extended period of time.

Is it always going to be that painful? If it is, I'm not going to complain. If this is what needs to be done to kill this cancer, then I'm going to do it. I don't have a choice. You knew this was not going to be enjoyable, Jessi.

She reinserted a different needle into my skin, trying to get it in the correct place. Once she pushed that mysterious liquid into the other end of the tube again, I tasted something odd. I was automatically relieved. I responded with, "Ohhh, that's much better." *It worked.*

Come to find out the first attempt was a failure due to her missing that special cushion area on the port. Because the needle wasn't in the port itself, she was injecting the fluid directly into my flesh. *That is why it was burning so badly. But this isn't the chemo. Is the chemo going to burn?*

Had it not been for the "odd flavor" when she injected the fluid, I would have not known she was injecting anything at all. It "tasted" very unique. Not exactly like citrus, but that is probably the closest thing there is to describe it. However, that's not why I classify it as an odd flavor. I say odd because it was not in the same way you taste and experience flavors of foods. I wouldn't define it was a "taste" because it wasn't on my tongue. It was a sensation in the back of my nose. Whenever I would exhale out of my nose, I would get a "sense" of something similar to citrus. It is very difficult to explain. It's not a taste; it's not a flavor. It's a sensation similar to tasting, but not quite tasting. It's a flavor similar to citrus, but not quite citrus.

She gave me "premeds" and explained that they were the medicines given before chemotherapy. They were to diminish the side effects of the chemotherapy. "The medicines are like a cocktail."

A cocktail? How ironic she's talking about drinking. She has no idea what the last few months of my life has been like.

"It may take a little bit to find the right cocktail or mixture of medicines that work for you, but the side effects of chemotherapy are not as bad as they used to be. We have a lot of different options to help you through it."

Well, that's the first good news I've heard in a long time. Do they have something to keep me from losing my hair? Yeah, right. I couldn't get that lucky.

The premeds consisted of a lot of medicines I wasn't familiar with. I was still worried about the concept of injecting some nasty concoction into my body. It was a poison. Would it have the skull and bones logo on the bag? It's common knowledge to steer clear of poison. Purposefully injecting a poison to somehow cure me still seemed off to me. I knew that the chemotherapy would kill the cancer cells, but I knew it would wipe out all of my good cells too. It killed. As much as I wanted to pretend it wasn't a concern, I, in fact, definitely did not want to die.

After about an hour of receiving my premeds, it was time for the chemotherapy. The nurse came in carrying what I assumed was additional bags of saline solution. She hooked them up to a machine that was attached to a pole. She pushed a lot of buttons and said, "Okay, I set the drip to be done in about two hours."

As she was getting ready to leave the room, I asked surprised, "That's it?"

She looked at me a little confused and said, "Well, let me double-check." She looked at her sheet of instructions and continued, "Yes, it says to set the drip to be completed in two hours."

"No, I mean, that's the chemotherapy?" I was looking at a seemingly harmless clear liquid in a normal-looking bag. It was clear. *A clear liquid. It doesn't look scary.*

"Yes, that's the chemotherapy." She pointed to the deceivingly innocent-looking poison.

Mom chimed in, "What did you expect, it to look green and bubbly?"

Dawn and Mom chuckled.

A CANCER MADE MESS

I sheepishly replied, "Yeah… I didn't know." I suddenly realized how silly that thought was. How carried away my worries had actually gotten.

"Well, the color depends on the type of chemotherapy. We actually do have some that are a bright cobalt blue," the nurse informed us. That statement made me feel a little better. My vision of it being odd, scary, and horrible—anything but clear—wasn't too farfetched.

After the nurse left the room, I sat silently staring at the clear poison slowly dripping from the machine into a long tube that was connected to my port and realized my life had just changed forever. The chemotherapy treatment had begun.

I'm officially a chemotherapy patient.

> *Fear gripped me, and my bones trembled.*
> *—Job 4:14 NLT*

18

Miserable Aisle

As we sat there in silence, we heard not-so-pleasant noises from other chemotherapy patients. One lady sharing a wall right next to us kept moaning in agony. Each time a nurse would go in, we would hear her adamantly complain about how badly her leg hurt. When they would try to rearrange her, she would cry out in pain.

There was a man on our other wall who kept vomiting and dry-heaving. Someone farther down the hallway kept coughing a nagging cough. *The nurse said that chemotherapy isn't as bad as it used to be? What did it use to be like? This sounds pretty bad.*

People were raising their voices in frustration. People were crying. People were in pain. People were *miserable*. Everyone was upset. Everyone was in turmoil. And I was right in the middle of it all. It was as if I was in the middle of misery aisle. *I don't belong here.* Looking back, that was exactly where I belonged. I was miserable, even if I didn't want to admit it.

I felt very lucky not to be in any one of their positions. However, I could not help but worry that I would eventually end up enduring the same suffering right alongside them.

Dawn had come prepared. She brought a variety of different card games, most of which I had never heard of, to keep us entertained. I was not up for any type of concentration, so I tried to mindlessly watch TV. All I could find was *Gangland*. I watched it briefly until I grew tired of watching dumb people make their own misery.

I started to feel angry and annoyed with the people on the show. *These idiots made poor decisions, and that's why they are in the bad situations that they are. They made their life that way. That's on them. What have I done to deserve the price I'm paying? Why do I deserve this? This is unfair.* After realizing that I was getting caught up in my thoughts, I decided a distraction might be a good idea. Cards, it was. The cards were fun. We actually laughed. I couldn't remember the last time I laughed.

While playing cards, I kept getting caught up in the tubes coming out of my chest. When I had to go to the bathroom, we unplugged the machine from the wall so that it would roll along with me. When trying to get out of the chair, my tubes would get caught on the arm of the chair. When trying to get out of the door, my tubes would catch the doorknob. There were so many cords and long strings of tubes coming out of me and that machine that it made it complicated to try to get anything done. I felt twisted—trapped.

About an hour into the chemotherapy, I started to feel nauseous. Dawn quickly told a nurse. They gave me some antinausea medicine. It helped; however, that first side effect put me in a state of fear. I sat there in expectation, expecting that I would become like my fellow chemo neighbors any second. I sat in fear, waiting for a horrible sickness to engulf my body.

Before too long, the nurse came in and said, "Okay, you're done!"

Time's up? It's time to go home? I feel tired and a little nauseous, but I'm okay. I'm okay. Am I really okay? I feel okay! Not great, but I'm okay! I'm not throwing up. I'm not in pain, am I? No, I'm not hurting.

After a few seconds of positive thinking, I started to become skeptical again. *It must be going to hit me later. It can't be this easy.*

Dawn, who lived in Missouri, came with us to Mom and Dad's to spend the weekend. My parents' house had a window unit for air-conditioning and did not cool my back bedroom very well. Being the beginning of August, it was hot. Hot *hot*. So my family set up a spot for me in my dad's man cave, "the bunkhouse." It was well cooled.

About an hour after getting home, I started to feel a little more drained and a bit achy. As time crept on, it worsened—quickly. I was suddenly exhausted. I felt as if I had a very bad case of the flu. I did not eat supper. I just wanted to go to bed.

My sister came into the room with an overwhelming amount of medicine bottles and started rambling off what they were for, when to take them, and what the side effects were. She had made it a point to ask the staff every detail about each medicine. I was appreciative of how she had taken it upon herself to take that on. I felt like it lightened the load on me immensely, one less thing I had to worry about, someone taking initiative and helping. *I sure do love her.*

I spent the weekend lying in bed watching TV. On regularly scheduled intervals, my sister would pop in, proudly carrying the box of medicines to distribute "the goods." By the end of the weekend she had written brief explanations on the bottles of what they were for and when I should take them. I appreciated it more than I let her know.

By Sunday, it was time for her to go back to Missouri and time for me to head back to my apartment to get ready for work the next day. Before we went our separate ways, she passed the box onto me. It was now my job. I was not looking forward to the responsibility.

It was extremely important to take the medicines on time. It was a particularly daunting task that I did not want to bother with. There were some medicines I had to take for two days before chemo, some medicines to take for two days after chemo, some medicines to take all the time, and then others to take when I had certain side effects. There was a lot. And the medicines to take two days before and after chemo were the most important. If I didn't take those, I would feel even more miserable, or worse yet, chemotherapy would be postponed. At that point in time, that honestly was not that dreadful of an aspect for me. I would have been ecstatic to reschedule a chemotherapy treatment, which is exactly why me being in charge of the medicines seemed like such a bad idea. *This important box should not be left in my incapable hands.*

I left my parents' house that day carrying the box of medicines to my car, feeling as though it weighed three hundred pounds. It was a lot to have it all on my shoulders, my responsibility. I felt lost, scared, and alone.

> *This is my command—be strong and courageous!*
> *Do not be afraid or discouraged. For the Lord*
> *your God is with you wherever you go.*
> *—Joshua 1:9 NLT*

19

The Promise

The next week, my childhood best friend, Jacob, came to work for my dad. Jacob did that now and then. He had a habit of working somewhere a while, growing tired of it, and moving on to something else. That was just Jacob. My family accepted him as a part of the family, and we all were happy to see him, especially during this time. Jacob was a lighthearted breath of fresh air to our stale sadness.

Jacob's own daughter had been diagnosed with brain cancer. She had surgery and underwent chemotherapy. She lost her hair. He had been there. He'd seen it all. Being around me, a cancer patient, was not anything new to him, which was comforting.

Everyone else around me was so shocked and appalled by the fact that I had been diagnosed with cancer that I was used to people treating me as if I was a freak of nature. I heard way too many times, "You are too young for cancer." So many times that I got tired of hearing it.

I even once received a full-on argument: "You won't get a hysterectomy. You must have misunderstood." Most people at work didn't know what to say to me, so they avoided me entirely. That was actually my preferred method of social interaction: none. I didn't want to talk to anyone about it, and I was tired of the same questions.

I had way too many interactions with the sad eyes, awkward hugs, and sighs heavy with sympathy. I was mostly tired of the fact that I wasn't able to stay in denial when people would call me out on it and ask me about it. I made every attempt to not tell people at work (except a limited few) what was going on to avoid even more conversations, but it didn't work. It got to where if someone came into the classroom I was teaching in, I would get anxious, worried they were going to try to talk to me about it.

There were a limited few, though, whom I did confide in. One of whom was Terry, who once grabbed our work calendar, sat down, and asked me the chemo treatment schedule. I explained the three-week cycle to her. She started marking the chemo days, all of which were on a Friday, with a cute Care Bear sticker. I smiled. I liked Care Bears from my childhood. I always thought they were cute.

My favorite particular Care Bear sticker was the one with the rainbow on his belly. When I mentioned that, Terry explained that a rainbow symbolizes God's promise to us. He promises not to flood the earth again. He promises to be with us. He promises to take care of us.

I didn't quite understand who God was at that point in my life. I had a misconception that He was a judging, noncaring, mean God. Terry started to show me that God was not what I had thought. She gave me a devotional, a Bible, and many hours after work, explaining to me who Jesus really was. She told me that Jesus was our Savior—our Lord. God is a caring, patient, loving Father who wants nothing but the best for us. I didn't quite believe that God could be as good as Terry was explaining as I had been raised with a very different perception of Him. Nonetheless, I listened to what she said.

Hearing about God didn't stop me being dumb, however. I continued to drink. I was a chemotherapy patient drinking. Heavily. Still with the same crowd. It helped me not feel alone. But mainly, it helped me continue to push down the feelings that once came busting through. I was determined not to let it happen again.

The next Friday, it was time for chemo again. Dawn came to meet us again at the cancer center. This time, it was the two types of chemotherapy on the same day. It was the same events as the first day. This time, my inflammation from the port placement had enough time to subside, so inserting the needle into the port went much smoother. Premeds for about an hour. The first chemotherapy lasted two hours. I felt about the same as the first time, tired and nauseous.

Then it was time for the second type of chemo. *Would this chemo be worse? How is it different? Will I lose my hair today?*

The second type of chemotherapy took longer. About three hours. I felt a bit more tired and a little more nauseous, but not too bad. Later that night, it felt like a bad case of the flu. Achy, clammy, nauseous headache. I spent the night in the bunkhouse with Dad. When Monday came, I went back to work—and drinking.

By this time, the kids were back from summer break, and I was teaching preschool again. On the classroom calendar, Terry had marked off two Care Bears, two rounds of chemo down. *Maybe I won't lose my hair. Two down, and I still have it. Mom said that Grandpa didn't lose his. She said that it might be hereditary that I keep my hair. Maybe she's right!*

The next week, Friday was yet another two-hour drive, but no treatment this time. I met with my oncologist. He did a CT scan and said that the CT showed some spots, but they were most likely pools of liquid that were still trying to absorb back into my body after the surgery. He instructed that I would have to go get a white blood cell booster shot the next day, Saturday. He set it up for me to do it at my local hospital, so that I wouldn't have to drive two hours to get the shot. *A shot? That will be easy. As many times as I've been poked already, that won't be a big deal.*

Saturday morning, I went into my local hospital and received my white blood cell booster shot. They injected it into my arm. It burned a bit, and it was sore for a couple of hours, but that was that. *No big deal.* My lower back was oddly aching, but I barely noticed. I made it a point not to notice. When Monday came, I went back to work—and drinking.

I found myself suddenly surrounded by Care Bears. Everywhere I went, stuffed Care Bears were being brought to me by everyone around me. Even students brought me their own sweet Care Bears of their own. I will never forget walking to my car to find the biggest fluffiest pink Care Bear sitting in my driver's seat (thank you, Carolyn). I was given plastic Care Bear figurines, books, blankets, clothes, the list goes on.

Each bear symbolized so much more to me than what people even realized. Every time I saw one, I was reminded of the story that Terry told me about God's promise with the rainbow, promising not to bring devastation again to His people. Granted, I wasn't dealing with a flood, but I was dealing with devastation. I oddly sensed hope and peace when I was reminded of His promise. Because maybe, just maybe, God was trying to give me a promise of my own.

> *Your promise revives me; it comforts me in all my troubles.*
> —Psalms 119:50 NLT

20

Confession

One particular time, the guy I had been seeing took me into his room, sat me on his bed, and started confessing that he was a horrible person. I knew what was coming, but I didn't really want to hear it. We were to leave for a concert within a couple of hours. I had already purchased the tickets and was needing the distraction.

When he finally got done heehawing and confessed that he had slept with another girl the night before, I asked emotionlessly, "Are you ready to go to the concert?"

He looked stunned and confused. He asked if I understood what he had done. I answered with a *yeah* and a shrug. He must not have been convinced as he started to retell his "tragic" mishap. By the time he was done re-explaining, he was the one saying all the lines I was supposed to be saying. He was telling me that he was a loser, and I deserved better. As I watched his charade, it dawned on me: he wanted his confession to cause me to break up with him. Let's face it, he wasn't the type to be by someone's side during a major life crisis, and he wanted an out. I couldn't blame him. I wanted an "out" from cancer too.

When I once again asked him if he was ready to get going, he started to get mad. After he yelled that he wasn't going to the concert, that was when I started to feel the panic start to rise. I started to feel something slipping away, and it wasn't him. It was me. I needed to go to that concert. I needed to feel like the old me again by doing the things I used to love to do. The concert was two hours away, and I knew I couldn't find anyone else to take his place before it was time to go. I knew, at that moment, I was about to do something that would be classified as the lowest of my lows so far.

I, the cheated, actually started begging the self-proclaimed loser-cheater to go to the concert with me. I mean straight-up begged—no dignity left here, folks. I had stooped to a new low and it felt awful. My self-respect and sense of morals had officially exited my life. I knew this was going to be one of those moments that I would want to forget about, push down inside where no one else would ever see. Yet, my need to go to the concert superseded any last hope of self-worth.

He threw a fit, insisted on me paying for everything, and ended up going. That's all I cared about, someone to go with me. I drove the two hours while drinking out of a pint of Wild Turkey. By the time we were at the concert, I was so exhausted we ended up sitting on the floor the entire time. It didn't matter to me; I was getting an escape from my normal life of turmoil.

The next week was time for my first checkup since starting chemotherapy. While I was sitting in the exam room, alone, covered by my blanket, I suddenly started to feel exposed. By that point, I was used to sitting on exam tables in nothing but a blanket as thin as tissue paper; it was not a sudden sense of modesty that made me feel so exposed.

For a reason unbeknownst to me, I finally started to feel bad about my poor decisions I had been making lately. The dumb ones. The rule-breaking ones. I felt guilt. I felt as if everyone knew what I had been doing. I felt embarrassed. Had they known and kept quiet about it so I wouldn't explode on them? They probably figured it was just my way of coping when, actually, it was the opposite. I was not coping. I was avoiding.

After about an hour of sitting alone in the examining room, my mother and sister started texting me, asking if he was in the room with me yet. They had been placed in the "comfy chair" room and were obviously growing impatient.

In the midst of the longest wait we had yet, which seemed like an eternity, my thoughts started pouring in relentlessly. *I feel horrible that I have been so stupid. I need to tell Dr. Johnson. I need to tell him what I've done. He said he wants to know anything and everything of concern. This is beyond concerning. I want to just be done with this. What will he think when I tell him everything I've done? Will he think I'm a horrible person? Ugh I don't want to tell him. I was not supposed to have intercourse. He told me absolutely no intercourse because it could damage or hinder the healing from the hysterectomy.*

Suddenly I heard his voice in the hallway. *Oh my gosh, that's him. I don't know if I can do this. Tell him all of it...*

I sat staring wide-eyed at the door, expecting him to come waltzing in while I tried to hurriedly decide whether to admit the last months' worth of bad decisions.

After several long seconds, the door had still not opened. *He's grabbed the chart off the door by now to see who is in here and should have been in here by now. Did he walk past?*

Time continued to creep slowly by. *Oh my gosh, I've never waited this long before. Go figure when I'm in here in inner turmoil, he takes forever to get in here. Just hurry up!*

The longer I sat, the worse I felt. *I shouldn't be so careless with everything. I act like I have nothing to lose when, really, I'm scared of losing everything. I'm so stupid. I've been acting so dumb. I'm a horrible person. I need to just stop. I have messed up so much, so big.*

As more time passed, the more convinced I became that I had to confess everything to him—the whole truth. *I need to tell him. I have to tell him. Tell him everything.*

Finally, the door opened. *It's him. Finally. Hurry, tell him before you lose your nerve.* As he was still entering the room, before he could even close the door, I blurted out, "I have some things that I need to tell you."

He must have instantly picked up on the seriousness of the issue as his pleasant smile quickly transformed into a serious look of concern. He calmly said, "Okay," and sat down to give me his full attention.

I started, "I have had some drinks lately." *Tell him the truth.* "Several drinks."

He sat, stone-faced. I was unable to read him. *Just tell him.*

"I have been drinking a lot lately," I said with a sigh. I felt an odd sense of release with that statement. A sense of relief. A sense of freedom.

I sat and waited a moment, hoping that he would interject so that I would not have to continue. He kept silent. *Ugh. He's waiting for more. He knows there's more.*

"And I had intercourse." Another pause. *He's still silent. Might as well tell it all now.*

"More than once," I said defeatedly.

He did not have the response that I expected. He was not appalled. He did not even seem surprised. He calmly said, "Is that everything?"

I started rambling, "Yeah, I think that's all. I just didn't know how to deal with any of this. And I started doing something's that I shouldn't have. But now I have found God, and I'm okay." I stated it with the sincerest look I could manage.

What does that even mean that I have found God? Have I found God? Am I okay? Why did I just say that?

As I was sitting there realizing what had just came stumbling out of my mouth, I wondered if I was trying to convince him or myself. He didn't seem to need convincing as he comfortably started consoling me by once again saying how this diagnosis would have turned his world upside down had it been him. He also explained that he would be able to see if any internal damage was done during the exam.

He completed the exam and reassured me that everything was as it should be and "healing beautifully."

Next thing I knew, I was talking to another psychologist. It was the same female who I had seen before, the same one who prescribed me antidepressants in the beginning, the same one who had consoled Mom.

"I hear that you may have some things you would like to talk to me about?" She had me in a new room with a young female student by her side.

Not really. I already told Dr. Johnson, and that's all that matters. Nonetheless, I felt obligated to tell her what the fuss was about. "I told Dr. Johnson that I have been drinking a lot, going out and partying, and having intercourse."

"Okay, are you in a relationship?" she calmly asked.

I wouldn't really call my current "boyfriend" a relationship. I've only been with him maybe a month. I know full well that this is not going anywhere.

Instead of explaining the situation, I gave a simple no.

That must have given her the impression that I was sleeping around with random men as she then asked, "Do you feel that your choice of having casual intercourse has been detrimental at all to how you feel about yourself? To who you are?"

I sat quiet for a moment and thought about that statement. She was probably pleased that I was actually giving something some thought, but I'm almost positive it wasn't the thoughts she had hoped for. She wanted me to really come to terms with how my poor choices were truly affecting my course of life. However, these were actually my thoughts:

> *How could that be detrimental to who I am? First off, it was the same guy. She said "casual intercourse," so she thinks I'm a floosy. Not like I was having one-night stands. Second off, even if I was having one-night stands, I still don't see how that could be considered detrimental to who I am as a person. I'll tell you what's detrimental to who I am—being diagnosed with cancer, having to endure chemotherapy, knowing that I am most likely going to die in five years.* THAT *is detrimental to who I am. Intercourse, though?*

After sitting there looking into my lap for maybe ten seconds, I raised my head to look her dead in the eye and answered with another simple *no*. I had much bigger issues to deal with rather than take the time to explain my life and my decisions to a stranger.

She looked a little shocked. That was obviously not what she was expecting to hear. The meeting ended shortly after that. When

I told Mom and Dawn about the conversation, Mom said, "Why didn't you tell her you have a boyfriend!" She seemed upset that I had let someone think I was sleeping around.

I said, "Because it's not really a relationship if there are no feelings involved. Yes, we are dating, but I don't care about him." That may sound rather heartless, as my mother stated, but it was the truth.

As I was leaving the appointment, I realized I felt *lighter*. Maybe the truth really does set you free. I no longer felt that there was a deep, dark secret hidden. I no longer felt ashamed of my poor decisions. I no longer felt weighed down with guilt. It was all in the open.

After that appointment, I decided to end all unhealthy relationships. With that decision, I stopped going out to bars. I finally ended the not-what-I-call-a-relationship relationship. I simply stopped hanging out with the wrong crowd altogether. I stayed in my small apartment with my cat.

With that change, I wish I could say that I started to accept having cancer. But I did not. I still did not know how to deal with what had been dealt to me. I continued to keep pushing my feelings downward. With the continuation of denial, the drinking also continued. When I was not at home with my cat, I was at my parents' house drinking with Jacob. Heavily.

*Turn to me and have mercy, for I
am alone and in deep distress.*
—Psalms 25:16 NLT

21

Branded with Cancer

I had been told by several sources that hair loss would happen around the third treatment of chemotherapy. They said it would fall out in the shower. It would come out in clumps—by the handful. The idea of losing my hair was very traumatic for me. I couldn't help but be consumed with the idea of becoming like one of the dead walking skeletons in the waiting rooms.

In my eyes, becoming bald would be the moment of no return. I wasn't just being labeled a cancer patient with a simple wrist band that could easily be ripped off. This would be more relatable to the agony livestock endure while being seared with a branding iron. I would be burned. Stamped. Marked. Branded. For all to see. It was cancer claiming that I belonged solely to cancer itself. I would no longer have control over any aspect of my life. Cancer would have full control.

People tried to console me the best they could. I never explained to them the feelings that came along with the fear of losing my hair.

"It's just hair."

Yes, I suppose it is what you might call, in a sense, disposable or renewable. However, it is not "just hair" to me. It is a part of me, of who I am. A part of my identity. I have lost so much already. I need my hair to hang on to, that last glimmer of who I once knew myself to be.

"Oh, hair grows back."

It may grow back, but I do not want to be bald for a second, let alone an hour, a day, or a month, especially not until all of this crap is over! It's not like it's going to start growing back the next day; it will prob-

ably take over a year before it starts to grow again. It will be several years before I have my normal hair length back. That's a long time to carry the label of being a cancer patient. Being bald is as loud of a statement as a loudspeaker shouting, "Yes! I do, in fact, have cancer!"

"You've lost a lot more than your hair, Jessi. This isn't that bad compared to what you've already been through."

Yeah, don't remind me, I know. This is unfair! I hate everything about this. Every single thing. Cancer has taken so much from me already, and I'm being forced to face the ugly fact that I very possibly could die. Very soon. I'm going to die a cancer patient. Losing my hair would take away my last sliver of hope to having a normal life.

"You are beautiful no matter if you have hair or not."

That's a sweet statement, but I feel that my hair is what makes me pretty. I've always been so proud of my hair. I've never even had short hair. Being bald is a huge change—too big of a change. A change that symbolizes that I am now a cancer patient, one step closer to looking like the walking skeletons in the waiting rooms.

"You can wear a wig. You could be like Samantha on *Sex and the City* and use it as a fashion statement. Lots of different wigs! Might be fun!"

That makes me feel slightly better, although it's still not my hair. It is just yet another thing that cancer is forcing me to do. Forcing me to get this chemotherapy, forcing me to get a hysterectomy, forcing my family to be traumatized, forcing me to lose all sense of security, forcing me to wear a wig—when does it stop?

My mother reminded me that my grandfather didn't lose his hair when he had undergone chemotherapy for his colon cancer. She explained that I might take after my grandfather and not lose my hair at all. That gave me tad wisp of hope.

Maybe I won't be branded with cancer. Maybe, just maybe.

> *The thief's purpose is to steal and kill and destroy. My purpose is to give them a rich and satisfying life.*
> —John 10:10 NLT

22

The Third Treatment

On September 2, 2011, the dreaded day had arrived—the third treatment. While receiving chemotherapy, I could think of nothing but my hair. *People keep telling me that I look fine. I won't after losing my hair. I'll never be the same. Please don't let me lose my hair, God. If you're up there, if you're there, please don't let me lose my hair. I don't want to lose my hair. I'll be losing the last part of me, of who I am. I'll be branded a cancer patient and end up looking like one of those walking skeletons. I don't want to die. I don't want cancer. I don't want to lose my hair. I don't want this.*

While being injected with the chemotherapy, I almost expected my hair to start falling out onto the floor right then and there. At the end of the treatment when I checked my hair's stability by giving a handful a little tug, I was relieved to feel my hair was still firmly intact.

That evening, I felt worse than the previous treatments. My stomach was hurting, my back was hurting, my head was hurting, my whole body was hurting. I felt like I could vomit with the slightest twitch of the hand. *Ugh, has the chemotherapy had time to build up in my system by now? Is that why I feel so miserable? Or have I caught a bug? Am I really going to feel this miserable after each treatment?*

While getting ready for bed that evening, I dreadfully brushed my hair, expecting to have bald patches afterward. I was relieved to see no more came out the normal few strands. *Maybe I won't lose my hair! Or maybe it takes a little bit...*

I went through the weekend hoping that I had inherited my grandfather's ability to keep my hair during chemotherapy, as my mother had suggested. *The doctors said yes, I would lose my hair, but how do they really know? Maybe I won't.* It had been suggested to me that I should cut my hair and donate it to a worthy cause. They told me that it would be an easier transition to go from long hair to short hair to being bald rather than just long hair to—*zap*—bald. I thought about it. But I did not do it. As selfish as this sounds, I wanted to hang on to it as long as I possibly could. After all, there was a possibility that I wouldn't lose it at all.

I was grasping at any last hope of keeping my hair, so much so that I didn't shower all weekend in an attempt to avoid the dreaded "your hair will fall out in clumps in the shower." I also avoided brushing my hair; I simply left it in a low ponytail.

After spending the entire weekend at my parents' house, Monday came, September 5, 2011. In the hustle and bustle of getting ready to go to work, I had almost forgotten losing my hair could be a reality. I was mindlessly brushing my hair, and midway through the first brushstroke, I noticed the brush seemed heavy. I froze immediately.

Brush still midstride, my mind started to play a fast whirlwind of every comment I had heard about losing my hair. *You are going to lose your hair...bald...fall out in the shower...after the third treatment...fall out while brushing your hair...fall out in clumps...you can wear wigs...you should have cut your hair...*

Without moving the brush, I stood in the bathroom holding my breath, staring at myself in the mirror. I didn't want to move. I didn't want it to be true. *Oh God, no. Please no. No, no, no! Please no. Don't let this happen to me.*

As my arm grew tired, I slowly finished the stroke. I fearfully looked at the brush out of the corner of my eye.

There it is.

A large amount of hair was spilling off all edges of the brush. I took a gulp of air and stopped breathing. Every muscle in my body tightened. My eyes grew large, and I turned stark white.

My hair. It's falling out. It's happening.

My...

hair...
is...
falling...
out...

Each word was slowly thought in its own state of turmoil and anguish.

My—no one else's, it's mine. That's my hair on that brush. This is happening to ME.

Hair—the one thing that is allowing me to pretend nothing is wrong with me. Everything else on my body is changed, scarred, or hurting. My hair is the only piece of me that is still normal. Until now.

Is—it is not an *if* anymore. It is a *for sure fact* that my hair is falling out. It is happening. Right now.

Falling—alongside each strand of hair that is falling, it feels as if a piece of me is being ripped away. I am literately falling apart.

Out—no more hiding. My secret is out. I can no longer pretend I don't have cancer. Everyone will know by simply looking at me.

> *I have told you all this so that you may have peace in me. Here on earth you will have many trials and sorrows. But take heart, because I have overcome the world.*
> —John 16:33 NLT

23

I Am Losing It

After that first devastating brushstroke, I stopped brushing my hair. Both hands firmly griping either side of the sink, I stood in the bathroom for a few minutes, trying to rein in some strength. I wanted nothing more than to fall into a heap on the floor and cry, scream, and bawl. *Not now. Not now. Not now. Do not fall apart. Got a long way to go. Crying won't help. Falling apart will only make it harder. Pull it together, Jessi. You have no choice.*

I looked at the girl in the mirror. *What has happened to her?* My mind wandered back to where she was a few months ago, before the diagnosis, where nothing was wrong with her. Where the only things she worried about seemed so small and insignificant now. It was such a short time period ago, yet it seemed so very far away. *That was a different person. It doesn't feel like me anymore.*

Staring at the girl from my past, I longed to be her again. *This is one of the last times that I am going to look at that girl the way she is right now. Tomorrow she will look different. She will be bald. She will never look like this again.*

After realizing that I had been in the bathroom for quite some time, I threw the hair still attached to my head in a low ponytail. I quietly carried the large amount of hair from that one brushstroke into the living room where Mom and Dad were sitting on the couch.

I held out the offending clod that symbolized more than just hair. I said nothing. They both sat silent, looking at me. Mom's face showed sympathy. Dad's face showed fear. Seeing their expressions made me want to collapse onto the floor and start bawling. I wanted to let my mother's sympathy comfort me. That familiar sympathy that always fixed everything as a child was not enough to fix this. This was too big. It wasn't a simple scrape on the knee.

Don't start crying. Not now. I have to go to work. I have to get out of here. I am going to fall apart if I stay.

I walked over to the trash and watched as the ball of hair dropped to the bottom of the trash can. *That's a piece of me, of who I am. There's nothing I can do to save it. To save me.*

I quickly walked out the door without a single word being said. I drove the thirty-minute drive to town feeling like I had just lost a piece of myself. I could no longer hold back the fear. *This is really happening. I am going to be bald. I have cancer. I'm going to die.* I no longer felt as if my life was simply a bad dream; I was wide awake. This was real, and it was in full force.

When I arrived at my apartment, I took the most traumatic shower I've ever had in my life. Still clinging to the hopeless idea of trying to preserve as much hair as possible, I attempted to be as careful as I could. I very gingerly wet my hair, but it didn't matter what I did. Every time I barely ran my fingers through my hair, large clumps came out along with my fingers. *Just barely touching a strand, and it's like it's giving up so quickly. It's letting go. I don't want to let go. Please don't leave me.* I felt a piece of who I used to be leave me with each strand. I was losing myself. My identity. My future. My dreams.

I attempted to shampoo, just the top of my head, but more and more came out. I skipped the conditioner, deciding that was a pointless effort and got out of the shower. I gently patted my hair with a towel. I grabbed my comb. *Here we go.*

With each stroke of the comb, a large amount of hair would fill the comb. It was excruciating, yet it was completely painless—physically. I would have rather it hurt. Pain from razor blades digging into my flesh might have compared to the agony I was feeling on the inside. *How can it be painless when I am feeling so much pain because of it! I am losing so much. My life is over.*

All the things that I had held so close and dear were falling out into a heap on the floor. As I looked at the large mass of hair on the floor (which revoltingly looked like a large dead rodent), my thoughts were slowly coming and going. *My hair is gone. It is leaving me. I will no longer have my hair. I will no longer be Jessi. I am losing it.*

I was not only losing my hair. I was losing my grasp on what I considered reality. I was losing the image of me being fine. I was losing the ability to act as if nothing was wrong. I was losing all of my dreams of my intended future. I could no longer picture getting married, buying a house, having children, watching them grow, having grandchildren, giving my parents grandchildren. Each dream was being painfully, yet painlessly, ripped away from me, one by one.

After finishing combing my hair, I was surprised to see there was still quite a bit of hair left on my head. It looked thinned down, but I wasn't bald—yet. When I went to work and saw all the looks of sympathy from so many people, I couldn't hold it back. It became more than I could bear. I cried. It was the first time they had seen me cry since my diagnosis. It was short-lived, however. I told myself, *If you fall apart, you won't be able to put yourself back together. You have a long way to go. Pull it together. You can't fall apart now.*

Despite the large clumps of hair falling out, and the bald patches that were sure to appear, I decided not to shave my head. I wanted to hang onto it as long as I could. *I don't want this to be real. I am not going to help this process. I do not like it. I want to keep my hair. I want to keep me. I am not shaving it. It can all just fall out piece by piece.*

As the week went on, I lost more and more hair each day. I had very thick hair; therefore, the process of losing it was taking a lot longer than I had anticipated. I continued to keep my hair in a low ponytail, trying not to disturb the hair follicles. Still there would be several long hairs noticeably hanging past the end of my ponytail. I would try to just pull those few out, but a handful would accompany them. Once a coworker came into the classroom and absentmindedly looked in the trash and noticed one of the many grotesque balls of hair. She instantly became repulsed and blurted, "WHAT IS THAT!"

Terry must have said something to her because she suddenly ducked her head and said, "Oh," and quickly left the room.

By the end of the week, I had several bald spots on the back of my head; it was getting to the point that it looked noticeable. I finally started to come to the conclusion that something was going to have to be done. *It is going to fall out piece by piece until there is none left. I am going to end up looking like some nasty person with mange with only a few long strands of hair left. Like that nasty Sméagol creature off Lord of the Rings. I am going to end up bald one way or another, whether I shave it or I let it fall out on its own. This is hurting so excruciatingly bad. Maybe if I just get it over with, the pain will be over.*

On my dad's birthday, September 9, 2011, I had my fourth chemotherapy treatment. Later that evening, Mom, Dad, Jacob, and I had a cookout at my parents' house under their front awning. Smelling the delicious food and looking forward to a small distraction from my inner turmoil, I took my first bite to only have utter and complete disappointment. *No—not my taste buds too.*

I took another bite. *Cancer is taking everything I enjoy in life away from me. I can't even enjoy my food now.* I had been told of the possibility that the chemotherapy would kill my taste buds. I honestly didn't think it would be that big of a deal. I thought it may have been relatable to having a cold. It was completely different.

I dropped the food back onto the plate in disappointment. I used to think I couldn't taste my food when I had a cold, but I realized the taste of the food was more "dulled" rather than completely absent. Now I understood what it meant to have no taste. I would not have known there was even food in my mouth had I not physically felt it inside my mouth.

I sat somberly and did not talk. Without the distraction of being able to eat, I was once again attacked by my relentless thoughts. *I feel like crap. I can't taste anything, my hair looks horrible, I have cancer. I hate it. I hate this. I don't feel like living. What's the point?* I felt anger starting to boil inside of me. *This sucks. Life sucks. All my hair is going to fall out. There is no saving it. I might as well get it over with. I hate it. I want it gone.*

A CANCER MADE MESS

Interrupting the casual conversation everyone else was having, I angrily interrupted, "Well, let's shave my head."

This is my command—be strong and courageous!
Do not be afraid or discouraged For the Lord
your God is with you wherever you go.
—Joshua 1:9 NLT

24

I'm Ready

They all three stopped talking and looked at me. I turned to look at Jacob, who was sitting in a lawn chair beside me, and said, "I want you to do it."

I did not want to make Mom or Dad bear any more hardship. I did not want to ask them to carry any more weight than what had already been thrown on them. And, well, Jacob was used to this losing-hair stuff. He shaved his daughter's head when she was losing her hair because of chemotherapy.

"Okay, I'll do it," he said lightheartedly. It irritated me that he seemed almost happy to do it.

"Now. I'm ready now," I said with a cold-stone face. *It has to be now. I'm ready now.*

"JD, don't you have some clippers?" Mom asked.

Dad quickly disappeared to look for the clippers. I started getting nervous.

This is it. This is the last time I'm going to have hair. I'm going to go to bed bald. I'm going to wake up bald. I'm going to go to work bald. It's time. Everyone will see me bald. Let's get this over with. It will be over soon. This torture will be over soon.

Dad returned carrying—nothing.

Did he leave the clippers in the bunkhouse? Does he want me to go to the bunkhouse to shave my head? I don't want to go to the bunkhouse. I want to do it right here, right now, outside. I'm not moving.

"Sarah, come help me look for them. I can't find them."

Mom quickly got up to help search. *What? They can't find them? They better find them.*

Jacob tried talking about something. I did not pay attention. Ironically, the one thing I had dreaded for so long suddenly had an overwhelming sense of urgency. *This has to be done right here, right now.*

Jacob picked up on the fact that I was not distractible and sat in silence.

They both returned with no clippers. Dad explained, "I think David took them."

They're gone? I can't shave my head? I can't get this over and done with? It took me all this time to finally get ready, and now it's not going to happen? Imagine that. Another thing gone wrong.

I gave an angry sigh. A*rrrgghhh! Nothing ever goes right! Why can't this be done already! I want it done now. I need it done now!*

They must have seen the rage on my face, for they all started thinking of solutions. Dad quickly said, "I bet Dollar General has some."

Relief flooded over me. *Yes! Go. Hurry!*

"They're closed," Mom said.

The rage returned. A*hhhh! I have to put this off for another day? Nothing ever goes right! I can't handle this!*

I started to cry. *I can't stand it. This is too much! I just can't take it anymore.* I sat there under the awning at my parents' house in utter defeat, sobbing. My family had not seen me cry since before my diagnosis (apart from the chemo-panic-attack). Dad looked uncomfortable and started squirming and left. Mom came over and started to rub my back. Jacob did not move; he just sat in silence.

I want it gone. I want it to be over. I can't handle this. I need to be alone. I got up, took a shower, and went where I could be alone: the bunkhouse. I sat there with my head down, looking at my lap. I ran the comb through my hair and got it caught in tangles. I pulled the comb hard. Out came a chunk. *I wish this was over.*

I combed again, harder—another chunk. *Why can't this just be over?*

I combed even harder—a larger chunk. *I can't handle this anymore.*

I yanked the comb harshly through what hair was left. Another large portion of hair came out. *I hate this! I HATE THIS!*

The rage I felt inside consumed me. The hatred toward my hair consumed me. Before I knew it, I was yanking my hair out with the comb by the handful. I could tell some of the hairs weren't quite ready to let go as they hurt. *Yeah, well, I'm not ready to let go either, but that doesn't matter, does it? It's all coming out no matter what.* The agony I was feeling on the inside finally had some "realness" to it with each painful yank.

The process consumed me so that I did not see Jacob come in. I did not know that he saw what I was doing. I did not know that he then ran out the door and raced across the yard to tell Mom and Dad that I was yanking my hair out.

Next thing I knew, Mom, Dad, and Jacob came rushing into the bunkhouse. They stood at the doorway in shock, watching me for a few moments. Dad walked forward and sat on the bed, which was a few feet from my own, and watched in silence. Mom stood beside my bed with tears streaming down her face and watched in silence. Jacob appeared as if he was in physical pain as he sat at the table and watched in silence.

Suddenly Jacob burst out of the room; he could no longer handle it.

"Honey, let me do it," Mom said. She came over and put her hands over mine, stopping me midyank.

I put my hands down, breathing hard from the effort I had exerted. The anger was still boiling inside of me. I sat, silent, looking down at my hands on my lap. My fingers were red from the force I was applying on the comb. *Or is that blood?*

Mom started combing very slowly, trying to gently get the knots out, which was an impossible task due to the fact that every time the comb touched my hair, it would automatically pull hairs out and cause a huge knot not only below the comb but above as well. *The only way to get the knot out is to yank it out.*

Mom, however, did not yank. After a few seconds, she stopped and emptied the hair out of the comb. I heard her sniffle. *She's crying. Because of me.*

She continued to slowly and gently attempt to detangle the endless knots. She stopped after several seconds again to empty the comb. I heard another sniffle. *She's taking too long! Don't stop and empty the stupid brush—just get it over with.*

She slowly started to comb again. *Mom is crying. Dad is sitting there in shock. Even Jacob left. And he's the one who is supposed to be used to this. This needs to be over. That's it. I can't handle it.* I snatched the comb back from Mom and commenced yanking. Mom sobbed loudly and left. She went outside to find Jacob on the porch, hunched over, bawling. They embraced each other and sobbed for several long minutes.

I, in the meantime, continued to yank my hair out. Chemotherapy had already started to take a toll on my energy levels; however, anger fueled me. Dad silently lay on his bed and watched me as I tugged away at my hair.

Finally, exhaustion hit me. I collapsed onto the bed and rolled over, facing away from Dad's bed. Right before I passed out, I managed to run my hand over my scalp to assess the damage. There were several very large bald spots. *This is the last time I'm going to bed with this hair. I hate this hair.*

> *He alone is my rock and my salvation, my fortress where I will never be shaken.*
> —Psalms 62:2 NLT

25

It's Time

Early the next morning, I was awoken by Mom coming into the bunkhouse proudly carrying a pair of clippers, stating, "I asked Gerry if she had any of Tina's old clippers." Luckily, our neighbor Gerry had a daughter who had gone through beauty school.

With a sigh of relief, I said, "Okay. Let's do it." *Finally, it will soon be over.*

Mom suggested that we shave my head in the kitchen on the linoleum floor for easy cleanup. *There isn't going to be that much to clean up, Mom. There's not much hair left.*

As I walked toward the house, I got a nervous feeling in my stomach. *This is it. I'm going to be bald.* As I felt an overwhelming sense of dread, I told myself, *You have to do this. It's time.*

I sat in the kitchen chair while Jacob and Mom were getting things prepared. *Here I am, ready to get it done and watch the clippers not work. That's just my luck.*

"Do they work?" I asked. Jacob turned them on. *Wow, that's loud.*

"Yep!" he said, excited. *This is hardly a situation to be happy about. Jerk.*

I sat and watched Jacob trying out different attachments on the clippers. He caught me watching him and smiled at me. *He's always been so cheerful and carefree. That's just who Jacob is. I'm glad he's here. It's relieving. Better than all the darkness that's been surrounding me lately.*

"Is it going to hurt?" I asked quietly.

"No, they won't hurt!" Jacob answered as if I had asked the dumbest question.

My anxiety level started to heighten. *I am going to be bald. It is time. How does he know whether it will hurt or not? What if he gets my ear? Oh no, he's going to cut my ear. My hair is going to be gone. I am going to go to work bald. Everyone is going to see me bald.*

"Okay, just don't get my ears," I nervously said as I cupped them with my hands.

"Why? It won't hurt," he responded. *Why? Did he just ask* why*? Because I don't want my ears cut, that's why!*

The volume of my voice elevated, "Jacob, just don't go near my ears yet—you're going to cut them! Just stay away from them at first!" *I'm not ready. I'm not ready. I'm not ready. Not yet. Not yet.*

Jacob turned on the clippers. My anxiety level skyrocketed. "Jacob! You're going to cut my ear!" I shouted over the noise. He brought the clippers close to my head. I ducked and turned and shouted in his face, "JACOB! Do *not* get near my ears, okay! You're going to cut my ear! Just stay away from my ears!" I glared the most threatening look I could manage. *He better wait! I'm not ready!* I did not realize, but I was referring to more than just him cutting my hair near my ear. I was not ready to lose my hair, myself, my identity, my dreams, my future.

As I turned back around in the chair, I immediately felt a very strong vibration on my ear. I screamed in horror. Loud. "Ahhhh!"

I instinctively grabbed the offended ear. I turned and gave him an opened-mouth face of horror mixed with rage. *That was it! I wasn't ready. I just wasn't ready! Look what he did! He got my ear! I told him not to get my ear, and now it's done.*

My mom loudly accused, "Jacob! You did that on purpose!"

That JERK! I lowered my hand to see the blood…yet there was none. *There's no blood? Wait, does it hurt?* As I was realizing that I was not hurt, Jacob responded to Mom's accusations with an honestly spoken response of, "Well, yeah, I did! I had to show her it wasn't going to hurt her, or we would have had to listen to her screaming the whole time!" He rolled his eyes with an exasperated sigh.

I started laughing. *He's probably right.*

Mom started laughing. We all laughed. I was very thankful for the humor. I felt better after the laugh. Good enough to handle Jacob shaving me bald. I did not cry. During the process of getting my head shaved, I actually felt almost relieved. *It's going to finally be over.*

My lightheartedness ended when I saw Mom picking up handfuls of hair off the floor and placing them gingerly into a Ziploc bag. *Why is she doing that? Is she missing who I once was too? I wish she didn't have to go through this.*

After Jacob finished, I went into the bathroom and looked into the mirror. I stood frozen, appalled at what was looking back at me. *Look at that…bald person. That looks nothing like me. I wish I could just go back in time to what I once was. What happened to that carefree girl that I once knew so long ago? Was it really that long ago? What has happened to me?*

I ran my hand over my head—my bald head. *Oh my gosh. I have cancer.*

It felt weird not to be able to run my fingers through my long beautiful hair. There was stubble left. The stubble felt rough, not soft and smooth like my hair. *I do not like this. I want my hair back. I want me back.*

> *Don't be afraid, for I am with you. Don't be discouraged, for I am your God. I will strengthen you and help you. I will hold you up with my victorious right hand.*
> —Isaiah 41:10 NLT

26

Exposed Secret

When Monday came, I went to my apartment before work. I found the wig that I had previously purchased. It was big, poufy, and curly. As I stumbled around trying to find the correct way to wear the wig, I felt a small sense of hope. *At least I have a wig. No one needs to see my bald head.*

After I put the wig on, I looked into the mirror and realized the wig was not me, at all. *I look like a brunette Dolly Pardon. I hate this.* I wanted my long straight hair. Nonetheless, I decided it was better than being bald and headed to work, teaching preschool. The day was horrible.

By this point in time, my hot flashes had become overwhelming. My oncologist had warned me on several occasions that my menopause would have more severe symptoms due to my body not having a chance to get used to the gradual loss of estrogen (the natural way). He was right on with the severity of the hot flashes. I had a hot flash at least every hour. Each was a head-spinning, inside-boiling, about-to-pass-out hot flash from hell. I had even more if I sat down too long and got up to move or if I became upset.

The wig itself was hot and annoyingly itchy. Every hot flash intensified the itchy and hot factor of the wig. It was unbearable. It was all that I could do to not rip off the wig and throw it in the trash. *These hot flashes are flipping miserable. It's a hundred degrees out, and I'm sitting here feeling as though my insides are boiling with a mass of hot, itchy, stringy, not-my-hair mess sitting on the nape of my neck and on top of my head. THIS SUCKS!*

An unknowing parent saw me and said, "Whoa! You got a new hairstyle!" in a not-so-impressed tone. I was embarrassed. She obviously did not care for the look on me either. *It's a new hairstyle, all right. She has no idea. Everyone keeps looking at me funny. I don't like this. I feel dumb.* It was at that moment that I decided I was not going to wear a wig again.

As soon as I got into my car to leave for the day, the wig flew into the back seat. *There goes my one ticket to normalcy. There is no hiding this. No hiding the fact that I am bald. That I am a cancer patient. That I am probably going to die of cancer.* I felt defeated. The one thing that had given me hope was completely out of the question.

The next day, I dug a scarf out of my closet. I decided that if I was going to have to wear a scarf, I might as well make the best of it. I matched it to my clothes, added some dangly earrings paired with a long pretty necklace, and went on my way. I felt better. This was more me. As much as I despised the reason, I had to wear a scarf; I decided to like the look. It was as if I found a new fashion accessory. I stood in front of the mirror and stared at myself before heading out the door. *My hair was keeping my secret from being exposed. Hardly anyone knows I have cancer—until they see me today. I feel so vulnerable. This is it. My secret is out.*

Despite the overwhelming dread, fear, and vulnerability I was feeling, I headed to work. I thought I had received funny looks the day before, that was nothing compared to the stares and nervous glances I got while wearing the scarf. *You think you're shocked? You have no idea how appalled I am with the fact.* None of the adults were brave enough to question me, but I later heard that several of my parents went to the office to inquire. While the parents may have been reserved, the kids did not hold anything back.

"Miss Jessi! What have you got on your head?" they would ask with a smile, assuming it was yet another funny joke, similar to ones I would play on them often.

"It's a scarf," I would answer as I tried to muster up a smile.

"How come you have that?" Their little faces were in amazement. Their smiles were growing larger, anticipating the joke.

"Because I lost my hair," I quietly stated with yet another forced smile.

Their smiles faded, and worry crossed their faces. "Where did it go?" Their innocence was warming.

"My hair fell out," I tried to say it as happy as I could muster, which probably was not very happy at all.

"Why did it do that?" they would innocently ask, looks of despair on their sweet little faces. They got closer to console me. Before I knew it, little fingers were exploring under my scarf.

"Miss Jessi is sick, and the medicine she is getting to make her better made her hair fall out," Terry, my wonderful aide, answered for me. *Thank you, Terry.*

"Miss Jessi, you're sick? I've been sick! I had to go to the doctor! Did you go to the doctor? Did you have to get a shot? My brother had to get a shot! Are you going to be okay?"

They were all asking questions, looking at me in amazement. The poor innocents had no idea.

"Miss Jessi will be just fine! She just gets to wear pretty scarves now! Isn't she pretty!" Terry answered. The kids all joined in on the morale booster. *I love you, Terry.*

That was that. The kids seemed content with those answers. I would occasionally get a few questions from them concerning what kind of sickness I had. After they got some simple answers, they would go on their way. I was comforted by the fact that the preschoolers did not whisper behind my back about my ailment. They confronted it head-on with such innocence. They did not look at me with pity in their eyes. They did not tell me the very well-known fact that life was unfair. They did not tell me I was too young for cancer. They did not look at me and wonder if I would die. They did not treat me different. I was still the same Miss Jessi to them. It was exactly what I needed.

> *He uncovers mysteries hidden in darkness;*
> *he brings light to the deepest gloom.*
> —Job 12:22 NLT

27

Whispers

After a week of wearing the scarf, the nervous glances from the parents turned into looks of sympathy. Pity. Sadness. It made me upset. *If only everyone had the perspective of a preschooler.*

A friend of mine gave me a cap for my head to make wearing a wig more comfortable. It was like a pantyhose for my head. It was a very thoughtful gift, which I appreciated very much. However, I could not bear to try it on with a wig. *What if this doesn't work? I can't stand to get my hopes up again. I'm bald. I'm bald, and everyone knows I have cancer now so what's the point?*

I started to hate going out in public. When I went anywhere, people would stare. Work, stores, restaurants, even being stopped at a stoplight brought stares from the cars next to me. I hated that. I hated the whispers behind my back. I hated the awkward side-glances. I hated the turn-around-and-look-at-her moments.

I don't want to hear people's silent thoughts about me through their staring eyes.

If someone was going to stare, just please stand in front of me and stare at me. Don't give those awkward side-glances.

If someone wanted to know my story, just please go on and ask. Don't whisper.

If someone wanted to point out the young cancer patient, just please announce it over the intercom. Don't point behind my back.

It was not that I wanted attention. On the contrary, I did not want anyone to know my story. I was a very private person. But it annoyed me how people would think that just because I was bald and sickly-looking that I was also blind and deaf. I could still see and hear how they were acting.

When they stare at me like that, what are they thinking? "Look at that poor lonely girl with cancer. She's going to die." I want to scream, "Shut your face! Stop staring! I'm not a freak show!"

One day, while checking out at Walmart, the cashier and I were both standing silent, watching her scan the items. Without missing a beat, without even looking up at me, she suddenly asked point-blank, "What kind do you have?"

I was shocked. *Someone without hesitation, without whispers, without stares.*

"Uterine Sarcoma," I answered.

She did not hesitate. She did not look at me with sympathy. She did not talk to me with the I'm-so-sorry tone. She kept scanning the items and casually said, "I'll be praying for you."

I responded with a heartfelt, "Thank you."

Thank you for not whispering behind my back. Thank you for not seeing me as a freak of nature. Thank you for not being scared of me.

> *Give all your worries and cares to God, for He cares about you.*
> —1 Peter 5 NLT

28

Devastation Hit

It was time for another round of chemotherapy. This time, I felt like I blended in with the "cancer crowd" that was waiting in the lobby. *I have cancer. I feel like crap. I'm bald. This is my life—the end of my life.*

When a nurse asked if I had taken my premeds correctly the two days prior to the chemotherapy treatment, I lied and told her yes. The truth was, I had not been taking my medicines correctly; I had barely been taking any at all. I knew it was a big no-no as I had been told that chemotherapy would be postponed if I had not taken them as directed. However, I couldn't find the willpower to care enough to take care of myself. *I'm going to feel miserable anyway, so what does it matter?*

And I did. I felt horrible after the chemotherapy. Even worse than the times before. I talked Jacob into playing cards while having some drinks that evening in the bunkhouse. After several hours, he said he was tired and wanted to go to bed. I, on the other hand, wasn't ready for bed. I found it hard to sleep with the steroids they were giving me. I begged him to stay up for one more game. Then just one more. Then another. In the wee hours of the morning, he fell asleep holding the cards in his hands. I looked over at the bed nearby and saw Dad passed out as well. I downed the bottle of liquor that was on the table and stumbled to my own bed.

The next morning, when something was said about the liquor bottle being empty, I blamed it on Jacob. Dad knew better. He went to Mom and told her his concerns about how heavily I had been drinking. I laughed it off when Mom told me about their conversation. The next night, I managed to talk Jacob into more card games and drinking. Monday came, and I went to work, feeling much worse than the weeks before. I stayed in my apartment during the week, alone with my cat.

As time crept slowly by, the same cycle of events continued as well: chemotherapy, card games, drinking, work. Eventually, Jacob started to grow tired of being harassed to play cards. He would complain more and more each time but continued to humor me. My drinking intensified, as did the side effects of the chemotherapy, each treatment leaving me feeling worse than the time before. Achy, nauseous, exhausted.

One morning, after another night of drinking and card games, Mom confronted me. "Jessi, I'm worried that the chemotherapy won't have a chance to fully work with you drinking so much. Drinking is hard on your body, and it is going through enough right now." I could hear the worry in her voice. Hearing her worried bothered me.

It didn't hit me right then. It didn't even hit me the next day, but as I continued to feel worse from the chemotherapy treatments, I thought about what she had said.

She's right. This chemo is leaving me feeling as though I've been hit by a truck. Why am I putting my body through even more trauma by drinking so much? And what if the chemotherapy isn't able to work at its best ability? If I'm going to have to endure this hell, I don't want it to be in vain.

Remembering how worried she was when she talked to me, I realized that I was not the only one hurting. My choices were not only affecting me, but they were affecting my loved ones. I was not giving it my all. I was choosing to not care about my drinking. I was choosing to not care about taking my medications correctly. I was choosing to not care about my treatments. I was choosing not to care about my life. After some contemplation, I realized my true feelings were the exact opposite. I wasn't purposefully being careless with my life. It was simply me being too afraid to face the facts. I finally made the overdue decision: *From this point on, I will start trying.*

With that thought, devastation hit. I was no longer able to stay in denial. In order to start trying, I had to admit that there was something wrong with me. I had to accept that my life had changed—drastically.

I abruptly ran out of the denial stage and vigorously leapt into anger. The unfairness of my hidden truth kept gnawing at me. I was full of resentment that I had been placed in the situation that I had. A life that I did not want was being forced upon me, and I did not like it. I could feel the anger seeping into my innermost being.

I was angry at the world and anyone in it. I was angry at myself. I was angry at my hair. I was angry at God. *If there is a God, how could he let this happen to me? I don't deserve this. I'm going to die a young woman, without even a chance at life.*

> *What is the price of five sparrows—two copper coins? Yet God does not forget a single one of them. And the very hairs on your head are numbered. So don't be afraid, you are more valuable to God than a whole flock of sparrows.*
> —Luke 12:6–7 NLT

29

Loneliness

I started to become resentful that I was stuck with the life that had been dealt to me. I became envious to see my friends having a normal life. My friends were carrying on with their lives while my life had come to a screeching halt. It was no longer my life. It was cancer's life. My whole life and everything in it had been ripped away from me with one diagnosis. I was full of anger and disappointment. I would look at people walking down the street laughing, having a normal day, and start missing my life before cancer. Everything looked different. Everything felt different. Life no longer looked like the carefree and happy place as I had always seen it. It looked dead. I felt that I had no hope, lost and alone.

The more time passed, the less I socialized with anyone, including friends, family, and coworkers. I was secluding myself from the world and everything in it. I just wanted to stay inside my little apartment, my safe place, my hole. Alone. I became lost within myself, trapped inside my inner turmoil—closed in, closed off from the world around me. There, alone in my apartment, I twisted between anger and fear.

No one understands what I'm going through. No one ever will. This is my life and my life alone. They aren't the ones who are sick. They aren't dying of cancer so young. It's just me. Alone. Completely alone.

Laveda Dawn stopped going to chemotherapy treatments as she had a full-time job, although she would call and text every chemo day. When Mom chose not to go to a chemo treatment because her dog was sick, Jacob went along for the ride. I couldn't stop the resentful thoughts while I drove the two-hour trip there and back.

I wish I could choose when I go or don't go to this. I'm stuck with this. It's not an opt-in-or-out kind of deal for me.

It wasn't long until Jacob left. That's what my best friend from childhood was known to do. He would drift in and out of my life, somehow always showing up when I needed him the most yet never seeming to stick around quite long enough.

Everyone around me is drifting off.

My doctor said that one of the most important factors of treating cancer is the patient's mindset. The patient has to do everything possible to keep positive and maintain a good mental state. He told me that I needed to find a way, as impossible as it may seem, to become stress-free. Yeah, right.

Over the course of months, my fun-filled life had turned into a nightmare. There was no bright side. There was only cancer. What the cancer was doing to me. What the cancer was doing to my family. What the cancer was doing to my future, or lack thereof.

I started to fall into the deepest, darkest part of my life. I came to the realization that I did, in fact, have cancer. I came to the realization that I was going to die. My life was over. At my funeral, I would look the same as I looked at that very moment. Sick and bald. My family would have a rough time losing me. That was the part that bothered me the most.

What if I do die? What will Mom do? How will Dad handle it? I don't want to leave them. It will be so hard on them. Too hard on them. I don't want to hurt them anymore. They have been through enough. I love them so much. I don't want to leave them. I will miss them. I don't want to die. If I'm in heaven, everything is perfect, there is no sorrow—but how? How will I look down at them and see them crying and not be sad myself? That's not perfect.

I gave up on life. I gave up on having a normal life. I gave up on being happy. I gave up on ever feeling healthy again. I gave up on me. I gave up on hope. I often told myself that I was going to die soon. I told myself that there was no point in paying those bills because I was going to be dead shortly anyway. I told myself that it doesn't really matter whether or not if I was happy because there was nothing to be happy about. I told myself that I was okay with dying. I told myself I was alone. I told myself not to get too attached to this world because I was not going to be in it much longer. I told myself there was no point in life. I told myself that I had no future. I told myself my life was over.

What I had accomplished up to that point in my life was all that I was going to get done. *I haven't even done anything yet. Is this really it? Was that my life? That's all that I got? I thought I had so much time. I remember when I was a little girl asking God to help me help people. I prayed to him that he would guide me to a place where I could make a difference. Did I? I haven't helped anyone but myself. What happened to my dreams? They're gone.*

I felt that I had been thrown into a dark pit and declared that I should rot in misery all alone. I felt that I was supposed to suffer. I thought God had forgotten me. I thought that God was what I had been taught He was as a child—too busy to care about me.

In reality, I did not have to be alone. My mother would have taken me in, in a heartbeat. So would my sister. I could have taken my sweet friend Terry's offer to stay at her house. She insisted several times that I shouldn't be alone in that apartment. She insisted that she wanted to help, if I would just let her. Oddly enough, when I was around people, I seemed to feel even more alone. Being around people was a harsh reminder that my life was different, uprooted, ripped apart. I kindly thanked her for being so thoughtful but declined the offer. I wanted to be alone. It helped my feeling of seclusion seem valid.

Despite my feelings of loneliness and despair, people showed they cared. I had a team of people rallying behind me as I was blindly pushing forward. My coworkers went above and beyond to help me through the process, covering my shift when I was too sick to work, bringing me food, giving me money, coming to check on me in my apartment, doing my laundry, hosting fund-raisers, among many more thoughtful gestures that I am forever grateful for. While in the hospital, I was given enough money from my grandpa to afford living expenses that I otherwise would not have been able to afford.

Then on two other occasions when I had bills due and no way to pay them, my grandma's church gave me generous donations. Friends at work sold bracelets, a local tattoo business had a fund-raiser, and there were tons of other people that gave generous gifts, cards, and meals. So many that I cannot name them all.

Even complete strangers went out of their way to make a huge difference in my life. People I had never met were sending me cards in the mail with handwritten scriptures and prayers. Others were sending me home-cooked meals. Countless others were participating in fund-raisers on my behalf. I would constantly be told of people, even complete strangers, who were praying for me.

Every now and then, among the stack of medical bills, I would notice a card addressed to me from a stranger. I felt a sense of wonder. *How are these people this nice to me? They don't know me. I don't deserve all of this kindness.* As I opened the beautiful card, I noticed yet another scripture handwritten inside. It touched me deeper than words can express. *So many people are going out of their way for me. Me. Little ole me. Who am I to deserve all of this kindness? All of this thoughtfulness? So much generosity?* As I started to consider the fact that maybe the world was not completely filled with darkness and despair, I wondered if there was some light in the world after all. *Is there a bigger force at work here? Is God talking to me through these strangers?*

I started listening to people when they spoke about God. I heard about God's love and grace from Terry almost daily. I was still not sure what any of it really meant, but I liked to hear about Jesus. It didn't make sense to me, but I could feel a difference deep inside of me when I would hear about him. It was an odd sense of comfort that I could find nowhere else. I did not go out of my way to seek God, but I kept listening.

One night as I was aimlessly flipping through the channels, I saw a young bald woman on a television show. I was in awe that she was brave enough to be trying on wedding dresses with her bald head completely exposed in front of thousands of viewers. Her name was Margo and I immediately started searching for her on the internet. I found she had a blog and started reading about her cancer journey. I felt connected to her in a way I had never felt connected to someone before. We had several similarities: age, career, prognosis, yet that's not why I felt so bonded to her. The words she wrote spoke to my soul. Her thoughts and feelings were my own. Her struggles and fears were the same as mine. I felt as though her and I were bonded with a strength beyond words. Finally, I felt like I wasn't completely alone. I decided I needed to speak to her. I had to. I was devastated when I find out that the woman I felt such a strong connection to had lost the battle to cancer just months after her last post. I felt it was a foreshadowing of my own future.

> *Even if my father and mother abandon me, the Lord will hold me close.*
> —Psalms 27:10 NLT

30

Trudging Onward

Despite the fact that I would have preferred to have stayed in my apartment the entire time, I continued to go to work. I needed the money. I needed the distraction. I needed the kids' innocence reminding me I was still the same person, Miss Jessi.

From the first week of school, one of the kids' favorite books was about a character "trudging." I had explained that trudging was where the character was so tired that he did not want to keep going, but he kept stomping sadly along even though it was really hard. Each time they requested for me to read the book, I was expected to give an impersonation of trudging, where the kids would get a good giggle. As time went on and the side effects of the chemotherapy worsened, I started to feel as though I had somehow morphed into the character in the book, sadly trudging through a difficult life.

Despite the fact that I started taking my medicines correctly, with each chemotherapy treatment, the side effects would intensify beyond the previous treatment, resulting in me feeling a little worse than the week before. I started to feel nauseous more frequently, despite the antinausea medications. My eye pain grew to the point that I could no longer wear my contacts, even though I was using the shockingly pricey eye drops. It was as if the meds seemed to become less powerful as the chemotherapy side effects intensified.

It grew to the point to where I felt as though the inside of my mouth was covered with blisters. I soon learned that spicy or hard foods were completely out of the question. I couldn't even eat peppermint without feeling as though I was scorching the inside of my mouth and esophagus with a torch. Eating ice while receiving chemotherapy during the first few months somehow oddly lessened the mouth pain. However, as time slowly crept on, it too faded in its affect against chemo.

I continued to lose all my taste buds after each double chemotherapy treatment, which was every three weeks. I would start to regain taste just in time for the next round of double chemotherapies. Each time I took a drink, it simply felt like a cold tasteless substance sliding down my throat. *I can't even drink water and enjoy it anymore. I used to love water.* The disappointment with each drink caused me to drink less water than I should have, which in turn led to dehydration. My doctor kept stressing the importance of staying hydrated during chemotherapy. It was hard to say the least.

My skin was extremely dry and itchy. Some days my hands would tingle and go numb. My legs would swell to the point that it appeared my ankles were nonexistent. My nails turned yellow, and I became extremely pale. The hot flashes were ruthless. It would start out as me suddenly becoming extremely thirsty; then I would feel nauseous and as if I was going to pass out. Then the heat came: an overwhelming and suffocating heat deep from within me. With each hot flash, I felt as if it was burning up the last bit of strength my body had left.

All of those mentioned discomforts seemed to fade once the real pain began to hit. After each white blood cell booster shot, I felt even more wiped out than before. I felt all of my bones hurt to the core. I felt as if I had been run over by a semi. But the worst part was the pain in the bottom of my spine. It felt as if I was being stabbed with a knife. I pleaded my case to my oncologist, and he explained that the pain in the spine is expected; and unfortunately, the pain is progressive—meaning, it would get worse each time. He also explained again that chemotherapy wipes out immune systems, which can lead to much bigger issues than just treatment side effects. I had already been catching every little bug in the "germ factory," a.k.a. preschool, so it was imperative to get the shots. *No choice.*

He was right. The shots grew worse each time. So much that I would dread them more than the chemotherapy treatments. After trying a few different pain medications, I found one that helped with the pain. My oncologist warned me about becoming reliant on the pain medicine; therefore, I decided to deal with the pain more than not and took the pain medication sparingly.

The only way I could seem to find relief was to sleep, but I had trouble sleeping. Not only were my thoughts running wild, but the steroids I was required to take made refreshing and restful sleep almost impossible. I would constantly wake up and stay wide awake for hours. I would wake up every night around two o'clock. I would flip through the channels and end up watching *I Shouldn't Be Alive*. The show took my mind off the hardships I was going through. I liked to hear of people who were worse off than I was. And there was always someone who had it worse.

At least I'm not being crushed by a large boulder on the side of a mountain. At least I'm not injured and dying in the middle of a hot desert. At least I'm not being stung by a huge school of jellyfish while stranded in the middle of the ocean. It could be worse.

Near the beginning of my treatments, the nurses had asked me to rate my fatigue. I had always answered with, "Yeah, I'm pretty tired, maybe a 4 or 5." As treatments continued, I longed for the days of me not understanding what the term fatigue meant. It was more than just being tired. I was tired, yes, always tired, but my body felt as if it was slowly losing its strength. Every muscle in my body screamed at me that they could not muster the strength by simply stopping to work, occasionally resulting in me dropping things or even falling. It got to the point where my family insisted on pushing me around in the provided wheelchairs at stores. If they didn't have wheelchairs, we didn't go there. As time went on, the exhaustion overpowered the steroids, and I slept. A lot. I took four-hour-long naps daily, which was a big change (prior to cancer, I hardly napped). The exhaustion forced me to cut back on my hours at work.

It was becoming physically impossible for me to do a lot of the things that I had always took for granted. Even getting up out of bed to go to the bathroom became a chore. I would be panting, feeling as though I had run four miles, and about to pass out by the time I got to the toilet. It's a good thing I had a very small apartment, and better yet, that I'm a female and sat down to pee because I needed that break. I remember a few times when I would sit on the toilet and see black spots spinning around me. My doctor later explained that it was because my body was straining too hard. *First the cancer took my happiness, then many organs, my hair, my dreams, my peace of mind—and now it's taking away my everyday routines!*

I hated it. I hated that I could no longer do what I wanted. I had lost all control of my body. When I would throw a fit out of frustration, my body would smite me, and I would end up more exhausted than when I started. I felt as if I couldn't win. I was sick of cancer controlling my life. I wanted to be done with it. I wanted to be back to normal. I wanted to be *me*. I felt as if there was no winning.

Eventually, I learned a few tricks to make life a little easier. If I bent over, I almost passed out, resulting in a struggle while tying my shoes. Therefore, I left my shoes tied all the time, leaving enough slack in the laces so that I could use them as slip-ons. I planned small things out in order to make the effort count as much as I could. If I got up to use the bathroom, I made sure to grab something to eat in case I got hungry later and filled another glass of water, even though I had a full one on the bed stand already. I broke bigger tasks, like showering, down into smaller steps, taking several breaks during the process.

Considering how tragic losing my hair was, it wasn't even the worse part of treatment. Nor was it the many side effects, exhaustion, and seemingly endless aches and pains. No, none of those physical side effects were the hardest part of treatment. The worst part of receiving treatment was the mental aspect. Accepting the fact that I was no longer in control of my body, in control of my life; witnessing my family worry endlessly all because of me; spending countless sleepless nights contemplating whether I was in the midst of my last days on earth, feeling lost, feeling alone—those were truly the hardest things to deal with.

There came a time where I wanted to give up. I was not sure what that exactly meant, but I wanted to do it. *How can I give up? It's not like I have a choice. There's nothing I can do with this situation. It's not like I started a project and midway decided, "Oh, I'm tired of this. This is too hard. I quit."* I don't have that option. But I still want to quit. *I just want it all to be done!* Done *already! I'm sick and tired of feeling sick and tired! If I could quit, I would quit right now!* I saw no point in living, yet I heard something inside me say, *Just keep going.* I was not sure where I was headed, but I kept going. Day after day. Appointment after appointment. Needle after needle. Treatment after treatment.

I couldn't see the light at the end of the tunnel, yet I refused to let the cancer have complete control of my life, although I feared that it already had. I decided to—despite all the exhaustion, aches, and pains—to keep trudging onward into the darkness.

> *More than that, we rejoice in our sufferings,*
> *knowing that suffering produces endurance, and*
> *endurance produces character, and character*
> *produces hope, and hope does not put us to shame,*
> *because God's love has been poured into our hearts*
> *through the Holy Spirit who has been given to us.*
> —Romans 5:3–5 ESV

31

The Memory

The chemotherapy was hard. The exhaustion was overwhelming, and the pain was unbearable. Despite those side effects, as time went on, I couldn't deny the most frustrating part to cope with was chemo brain. Large chunks of time and important events are still missing from my memory. My short-term memory especially struggled horribly. My family tells me that I would forget and repeat things time and time again—small things, big things, all things. My mind wasn't "my" mind anymore. It was cancer's. I had always considered myself to be a fairly intelligent individual, breezing through classes, not having to study. To lose control of my own mind, the one thing that I had felt that cancer couldn't touch, was devastating. Hearing someone close to me laugh at me dismissively when I tried explaining that I was having chemo brain made me realize how misunderstood I really was. How misunderstood chemotherapy was. How misunderstood cancer was.

I often found myself struggling to finish sentences, not being able to find the correct words. Most of the time, I would have them on the tip of my tongue and not be able to say them. I would mix up words in sentences. For example, it would come out as "the caught dog the ball" instead of "the dog caught the ball." People would look at me funny and watch in silence as I stumbled around with my words. It was not only irritating but also embarrassing.

I remember things here and there in that time of my life—mainly the worst parts. The pain, the big scares, the long hours of driving, the exhaustion, people's lack of understanding. But there is one memory that stands out from the rest, one memory that is different.

I suddenly feel as though I'm being lifted upward and fast. I'm scared, terrified actually. Then oddly, the fear suddenly disappears. I somehow feel very at peace. Words actually can't describe how wonderful I feel. No more pain, no more worry, no more sadness. I felt completely and utterly alive and amazingly happy. I look above to see where I'm going, and I see light—the brightest light I've ever seen—yet it doesn't hurt my eyes. Soon the brightness surrounds me, and the sense of being lifted is gone.

I look straight ahead of me and notice to the left there is a tall man standing dressed in white robes. His right arm is outstretched, inviting me to him. I slowly walk toward him and notice his peaceful smile. There is something on the other side of him, but I cannot make it out. When I get to him, he pulls me in to his side, and I automatically rest the left side of my face against the right side of his chest. He wraps both arms around me in an embrace. For the first time since my diagnosis, I feel safe.

Was it a dream? Did I die in my sleep? I don't know. One thing I do know is that was Jesus. I felt it in my innermost self. I either dreamt or had a real-life experience, but either way, Jesus was real. My thoughts played the same loop of confusion for days, months, even years.

I put my head on his chest? That's kind of odd—for me. To just have that as an automatic response. With no hesitation. It was so out of character for me, yet it felt so natural and wonderful. He talked to me. What did he say? No matter how hard I try, I can't remember what he said. But I do know without a doubt that we had a conversation about something—what was it? Did he mention something about my future? I have a future. Maybe he said I have a choice. No, maybe he said I have a choice of a future. Maybe he said that I have a journey in front of me, and it's not my time to die. Maybe he said all of those things? Maybe he said none of them. But we did talk about something for sure. I wish I could remember.

All I know is, for the first time since my diagnosis, I finally felt a sense of peace, comfort, love, *hope.*

> *I am leaving you with a gift—peace of mind and heart. And the peace I give is a gift the world cannot give. So don't be troubled or afraid.*
> —John 14:27 NLT

32

Turn of a Page

I had recently been given several resources on God: a Bible, a Bible translation, and a devotional. I accepted the gifts graciously but did not really know where to start. I had never read the Bible or any literature on God for that matter. I expected the Bible to be full of stories of how wonderful life was, sunshine and butterflies all the way around. Feeling as though my life was more similar to a dark, lonely pit, I was honestly not looking forward to reading about how amazing other people's lives were.

One evening, while I was sitting alone in my apartment, I opened the Bible to a random page and was a bit surprised at what I read. It was not about how wonderful life was, nor was it about how fantastic it was to be alive. Rather, it was about a person who was suffering. Suffering badly. Feeling as though God had turned his back on him—alone, in the darkness, in pain.

> Lord, you are the God who saves me;
> day and night I cry out to you.
> May my prayer come before you;
> turn your ear to my cry.
> I am overwhelmed with troubles
> and my life draws near to death.
> I am counted among those who go down to the pit;
> I am like one without strength.
> I am set apart with the dead,

A CANCER MADE MESS

> like the slain who lie in the grave,
> whom you remember no more,
> who are cut off from your care.
> You have put me in the lowest pit,
> in the darkest depths.
> Your wrath lies heavily on me;
> you have overwhelmed me with all your waves.
> You have taken from me my closest friends
> and have made me repulsive to them.
> I am confined and cannot escape;
> my eyes are dim with grief.
> I call to you, Lord, every day;
> I spread out my hands to you.
> Do you show your wonders to the dead?
> Do their spirits rise up and praise you?
> Is your love declared in the grave,
> your faithfulness in Destruction?
> Are your wonders known in the place of darkness,
> or your righteous deeds in the land of oblivion?
> But I cry to you for help, Lord;
> in the morning my prayer comes before you.
> Why, Lord, do you reject me
> and hide your face from me?
> From my youth I have suffered and been close to death;
> I have borne your terrors and am in despair.
> Your wrath has swept over me;
> your terrors have destroyed me.
> All day long they surround me like a flood;
> they have completely engulfed me.
> You have taken from me friend and neighbor—
> darkness is my closest friend.
>
> (Psalms 88 NIV)

I was shocked. I stared in disbelief. I felt that every single verse somehow spoke to me, to the innermost part of me—a youth suffering, close to death, alone, abandoned, in agony, set apart with the dead. It truly spoke a sad but very real part of life: despair.

How could the Bible be speaking directly to how I felt? How could I have opened the Bible to that exact spot talking about despair? What's the chances of that? Out of the thousands of pages, here I was, landing on something that was meant for me. I was utterly amazed.

As I read it again, I found myself relating more and more to the overwhelming sadness that these scriptures portrayed. Hearing that someone had suffered so badly such a long time ago much like I was feeling at that very moment gave me an odd sense of comfort. Kinship maybe.

The more I read them, the more I realized the purpose of me finding those scriptures. It wasn't a mere coincidence. It was a message. God was sending me a message. He was telling me he understood my suffering. He was there with me through it all, right beside me through the sleepless nights, guiding the nurse's hands with each needle poke and carefully counting each and every hair that fell to that bathroom floor. God was there—feeling the torment, pain, and suffering, just as I was.

The scriptures immediately following Psalm 88 were once again a bit of a surprise to me. The sadness and despair that I was hearing was suddenly replaced with something quite different. There was a message beyond the suffering, and it was an even more profound message after the sadness and despair. It was a message of hope, strength, and comfort.

I was a bit confused as to how someone could change their outlook so suddenly. *Am I missing something?*

I read the scriptures again:

> Once you spoke in a vision,
> to your faithful people you said:
> "I have bestowed strength on a warrior;
> I have raised up a young man from among the people.
> I have found David my servant;
> with my sacred oil I have anointed him.

> My hand will sustain him;
> surely my arm will strengthen him.
> The enemy will not get the better of him;
> the wicked will not oppress him.
> I will crush his foes before him
> and strike down his adversaries.
> My faithful love will be with him,
> and through my name his horn will be exalted.
> I will set his hand over the sea,
> his right hand over the rivers.
> He will call out to me, 'You are my Father,
> my God, the Rock my Savior.'
> And I will appoint him to be my firstborn,
> the most exalted of the kings of the earth.
> I will maintain my love to him forever,
> and my covenant with him will never fail.
> I will establish his line forever,
> his throne as long as the heavens endure."
>
> (Psalm 89 NIV)

God, that's what I'm missing—it's God. That's it.

I realized that I had actually made little to no effort to include God in my journey. When I had received the call with the diagnosis, I didn't seek God for hope. When I was terrified on my first chemo day, I didn't ask for strength. When I would spend countless sleepless hours worrying, I rarely turned to God for comfort. I had always thought God was too busy to be bothered by me, yet here was a message from God himself explaining that he can be the one giving hope, strength, and comfort. I was unsure how to go about it, and I was honestly even more unsure as to whether or not I deserved it.

I knew that God was all too aware of how I had made some not-so-godly choices within the last few months. Yet to imagine that I had a God who loved me enough to look past my many failures to reach down and pull me closer to Him was the beginning of me learning who God really was.

JESSICA BELL-ALVAREZ

*For the Song of Man came to seek
and save those who are lost.*
—1 Corinthians 15:18 NLT

33

Brian

The long journey of being diagnosed and treated for cancer was finally coming to an end. With only about a month left of treatments, I felt as though there was finally a light at the end of the long, dark tunnel. At last, there was something to look forward to rather than to dread. The end date was in sight, and I could feel the anticipation mounting.

My anxiousness to finish the chemotherapy treatments came to a screeching halt when a chemotherapy treatment was postponed. My heart rate had been gradually growing faster, becoming such a concern that they had done several EKGs through the course of the treatments. It finally came to a point that my oncologist said there was no other option but to let my body rest for a week. We would pick back up where we left off the following week. It wasn't skipping a treatment; it was postponing it; meaning, my end date had just been pushed out another week.

The phone call left me feeling devastated. I had allowed myself to get my hopes up about something, for the first time in a long time, to only be let down once again. It was disheartening, to say the least. I was so physically, emotionally, and mentally exhausted. I was afraid I couldn't handle the delay—the disappointment.

During that week off, an unusual number texted me asking for my dad's number. From that one simple text, I had an odd sense of who it was. *This is him. I can feel it. Do I answer?* I couldn't remember the last time I had heard from him, my life before cancer seemed so far away. Instead of ignoring the text as I had done the many times before, I decided to ask, "Who is this?"

"You don't want to know," was the quick response I received.

Yep, it's Brian, all right.

Brian may have been correct in that statement merely a few months ago. I had been anti-Brian for some time. However, for some odd reason, I had been reanalyzing our broken relationship during my week off chemotherapy. Brian and I had a serious relationship which lasted several years and ended right before my diagnosis. Looking back, the immaturity of both of our actions was quite clear. As the week had progressed, I had even surprisingly started to remember some good times together rather than just the negative. He had a great sense of humor, a sweet soul, and despite his difficulty at expressing it, he had a soft heart. With my obvious inability to cope and express my own feelings of what I was currently going through, was I really that different?

"Hi, Brian," I replied.

"Hi." He followed up that simple text with a phone call. He had heard about my diagnosis. After a brief discussion about my cancer, he must have picked up on the heavy cloud of sadness that had been hovering over me for some time as he made me do something he had always been so good at, something I hadn't done in a very long time: Brian made me laugh. It felt good.

He wanted to see me. I warned him I looked much different. He insisted he didn't care what I looked like. I was nervous about what he would think about my bald head that was hidden under a scarf. I also had gained at least fifty pounds since he had last seen me.

The first thing out of his mouth when he saw me was, "You still have those beautiful eyes." *That's about all that's the same about me.* It hadn't even been a year, yet so many things had happened. So many things had changed. I had changed. I was no longer the same Jessi. My life had been turned upside down, and I felt as though I was grasping onto the edge of a very steep cliff, trying desperately to hang on. *He has no idea who I am anymore.*

Brian started to share some of his trials he had endured during our time apart. The last year had been pretty rough on him too. It brought a new sense of maturity to his demeanor. As our reunion was coming to a close, I couldn't help but think, *Well, this is the last I'll hear of him. Who wants to talk to a cancer patient, someone who is going to die shortly?* Yet he did. Over the next couple of weeks, he continued to keep in touch. We gradually started to see each other more often, with me always wearing a scarf, trying to cover my insecurity.

On one occasion, in particular, I had agreed to meet him at his house to help him study for a contractor exam he had coming up. I wasn't quite sure why he had asked someone with chemo brain to help him study as I was sure I wouldn't be much help. As I grabbed the textbook and took a seat, I felt a sense of panic start to rise as the scarf got caught on the book and started to slide off my smooth bald head. My biggest insecurity was on the verge of being exposed. I immediately grabbed for it, trying to keep my security blanket in place. Brian saw the panic on my face and witnessed my desperate attempt to keep it hidden. He immediately came over and grabbed the scarf off my head. In the time it took me to realize what had just happened, he had tossed the scarf onto the floor while strongly declaring, "You don't need that."

Embarrassed, I awkwardly sat, silent, waiting for him to decide otherwise and hand me back the scarf. Instead, he slowly bent over and kissed my bald head. I couldn't hold back the tears. Here was Brian, storming in and throwing my sensitivities to the side, literally. No hesitation, no tiptoeing around the issue, just busting right through to confront it head-on. Yet amidst his abruptness, he gently and lovingly let me know that he was supportive, accepting, and still very much in love with me. That was Brian, and that's exactly what I needed, as uncomfortable as it was.

> *And we know that God causes everything to work together for the good of those who love God and are called according to his purpose for them.*
> —Romans 8:28 NLT

34

In Over My Head

As time passed, the last chemotherapy treatment finally came and went. Friends helped celebrate by surprising me with Care Bear cupcakes. They were topped with my favorite pastel colors and adorable Care Bear toppers. *Look, they are bright, cheery, and happy—everything I used to be.*

Despite the relief of being done with chemo, the good scan results, and the celebrations of those around me, it didn't feel "over" to me. What had happened to me was not something I could just drop and forget. The horrible statistics kept replaying in my mind: I had less than a 20 percent chance of living another five years. I still felt as though I had a death sentence looming over my head while people were expecting me to snap back to the old Jessi, the happy Jessi.

Everyone is acting like I crossed some invisible finish line, and it's time to go back home now. They have no idea. There is no going back. Too much has happened.

Throughout the next several months, I found myself in a constant state of fear. With each new ailment, no matter how big or small, I was terrified it was cancer coming back to finish the job. *Was that bump there? Why does my wrist always hurt? Why am I having trouble breathing? Is that a discoloration? I never noticed that lump before.* I underwent countless additional tests, each coming back showing I was fine. Instead of feeling relieved with each reassurance, I oddly became more anxious. I felt as if I was on a hunt for a needle in a haystack, a nasty needle that needed to be eradicated, yet it kept hiding from me. There was nothing I could do but wait—wait for it to rear its ugly head.

After one particular test that concluded no cancer could be found, I noticed Mom was as downtrodden as I was about the test result. As we sat at a restaurant, both feeling defeated, I asked out loud, "What is wrong with us? The test showed no cancer. Did you want it to be cancer?"

Mom quickly answered, "No!"

"Then why are we so upset? We should be happy." Yet we weren't.

Even after realizing that enough time had passed to where I knew I should be moving forward, my paranoia continued to haunt me. I couldn't seem to shake the feeling that something horrible was about to happen—again.

What if I try to start my life only to get my hopes and dreams ripped out from underneath me again? I can't handle another disappointment. Not again.

What should have been the past was still feeling very real and relevant. I felt stuck.

Me being stuck in the past was an issue when I had someone right beside me wanting to move forward. Brian and I had moved into my small apartment together. In the midst of me being stuck in self-sorrow, Brian was there, accepting me for who I was. I hadn't even given myself that same courtesy, yet he was willing to look past the insecurities, past the fear, and past the cancer.

Despite his positive outlook and ability to move forward from what had happened, I was the complete opposite. I was mad that I would have to deal with the fear of cancer the rest of my life. I was angry that I no longer knew who I was. I was irate at the unfair hand I had been dealt. I felt torn apart at the seams, with anger the only thing strong enough to hold me together.

I morphed into a ball of rage, and Brian took the brunt of it. Often during my rants, I would tell him how he could never understand the feeling of fear I was living in constantly, what it was like to know that I was just waiting for cancer to return to kill me off. Most of the time, Brian would bite his tongue and let me rant and rave.

However, during one heated exchange, he yelled at me, "Well, you're not dead yet!" That made me even more irate.

He has no idea what I'm going through!

After things cooled down, he later asked, "How do you think it makes me feel to hear that you're so ready to die?"

I sat silent. *Ready to die? Is that what I have been acting like? Sitting around expecting cancer to return to kill me, I guess, is me accepting death. I never thought of it like that. But the truth is, I don't want to die.*

He continued, "I don't want to think like that because I don't want you to die." Hearing his heartfelt truth made me realize I hadn't really thought about his perspective at all. All I had thought about was me and my messed-up life, not the effect my harsh words or negative state of mind had on Brian.

Someone once asked Brian, "Why do you stay with her?"

Brian responded with, "Because I have faith she will get better." When he told me the conversation, I was a bit taken back. Not because of someone questioning my horrible behavior—I knew I was a mess—but because of his faithful response. *How can he be so positive and hopeful?* He had so much faith I would get better, yet…did I have faith? Did I see myself getting better? Did I see a future?

Brian clearly had a vision for a future, a future that included me. He started to make a few suggestions. The first was that I go to therapy. The idea of sharing my experience with a complete stranger who wouldn't understand what I had been through was not appealing. I had worked so hard to push down all the emotions and cram them all into a box hidden deep down inside. It would only take one little lift of the tightly closed lid for all of it to come rushing forward in an explosive spew. It would overwhelm me, overtake me. I would fall apart from the inside, unable to put myself back together again. I couldn't go talk to a therapist; it simply wasn't an option. I pretended to ignore the suggestion.

The next change he suggested was us getting a bigger place. I felt a sense of panic rise from deep within me. During the most tumultuous time in my life, the one steady, reliable, and constant thing had been that small yet quaint studio apartment. It was my safe haven, my little hole away from the world.

Why does he want to change everything? Things are fine just the way they are. I'm not going to therapy, and I'm not moving.

A few more months passed by, with Brian making suggestions of change and me clearly not wanting to make them. During one particularly irrational blowup, I went a step above and beyond in my outbreak. In anguish, I grabbed a large knife and fell to the floor and considered stabbing myself. The knife felt out of place in my hand, as though it didn't belong. Brian rushed over and took the knife from me. The despair continued, and in rage, I broke his TV. A neighbor must have been disturbed by the noise as the police came knocking on my door. By that time, Brian had left to spend the night elsewhere. After hearing a bald woman's confession to how a broken TV ended up on the porch, they didn't stay long. I was glad as I felt completely mortified.

I can't believe I broke his TV. I can't believe I got the cops called on me. Why did I grab that knife? I wasn't really going to stab myself, was I? I can't believe I've allowed myself to stoop to this level. Who does this? I know better than to act like that.

I literally felt like I lost all control. It's like I went crazy. What happened?

"WHAT'S WRONG WITH ME!" I screamed at myself in the mirror, tears streaming down my face.

Brian is gone. I've made a jerk of myself—big-time. He will never talk to me again. He's finally realized that I'm too broken to be repaired. I've ruined everything. My life is a horrible mess.

As I stood looking at myself in the mirror, I realized my life wasn't the only thing that was a mess. I myself was a complete and utter mess. My life was supposed to have been back to nonmess status with treatments being over, yet I was the biggest mess I had ever been. I had always been the levelheaded and reserved one. Never the type of person to be this unstable. I had gone from one extreme to another: a closed-off, hide-all-emotions type of person to a literally crazy lady filled with pure rage—and now regret. I felt shattered. My life had come crashing down around me and resulted in me being broken into a thousand pieces. I was too far gone. Too many pieces of myself were scattered and crushed that I would never be able to put them back together again. I was in over my head. It was too late. I was too far gone to fix.

    I curled into a ball on the cold bathroom floor and lay there alone, bawling a gut-wrenching cry. The harsh words I had screamed at Brian were still floating in the air. I could still hear the sound of his TV breaking. I could still feel how out of place the knife felt in my hand. Out of sheer desperation, I finally admitted through a sob, "I need help."

> *No power in the sky above or in the earth below—indeed, nothing in all creation will ever be able to separate us from the love of God that is revealed in Christ Jesus our Lord.*
> —Romans 8:39 NLT

35

Intake

I made it through the night and called Brian the next day. He came over, and we had a long talk. After such a horrific fight, he amazed me by being calm and supportive. "You need to see a therapist. They will know how to help you." I could hear the tenderness in his voice as he explained how the therapists are trained to help people like me. His niceness toward me after I had acted so horribly made me feel even worse—yet also made me love him all the more.

That week, my hands were shaking as I made the call to the local mental health clinic. It was hard overcoming the fear of someone analyzing me and telling me how messed up I was. I knew I was horrible and wasn't looking forward to a stranger pointing out my failures. However, the hardest part was facing the fact that I would have to relive the events over the last year, to stir up all the emotions I had tried so very hard to push down and hide. *I'm barely holding it together right now. If I open up, I will fall apart and not be able to put myself back together again.*

The next week, as I walked into the building, my nerves were at a peak. Ashamed and embarrassed that I didn't have it all together, I kept my head down and my voice quiet during check-in. Afterward, I sat nervously in the waiting room. I contemplated leaving, just walking out. *I am beyond the point of being able to be fixed. There is no hope for me. These people have never seen anything quite as messy as me. I am going to be the oddball "trouble case."*

"Jessica Bell," a dark-haired middle-aged man called my name. Keeping his eyes on his clipboard, he barely looked at me as he led me into a small comfortable room. He explained that he was not my therapist; he was simply going to complete what they called an *intake*. This was the first step to figure out which therapist would best suit my needs. Without glancing from his computer screen, he started asking all kinds of generic questions while typing the answers into the database. I assumed I was just another number on his list of to-dos as he seemed a bit distant, maybe in a hurry? Or was it boredom? The generic questions continued for at least thirty minutes when, oddly, he asked me to spell an eight-letter word backward. Afterward, he replied, "Wow, that was fast."

With his comment, I realized it had been quite a while since I had actually felt intelligent. Losing several mental abilities due to chemo brain was something I still found myself struggling with. I was constantly finding myself stumbling over sentences and searching for words that lingered just at the tip of my tongue during normal, everyday conversations. *Maybe the chemo brain is finally wearing off. Maybe I'm starting to get me back.* In the midst of daydreaming about the old days where I actually felt intelligent, I was abruptly pulled back to reality when he finally asked, "What are you seeking therapy for?"

Here it is. I felt my nerves start to rise. *Don't get into it with him. Don't waste your effort explaining everything to this guy. He isn't going to be the one to help you. Besides, if you tell him how much of a mess you really are, he might say, "We can't help you."*

I swallowed hard, took a deep breath, and answered, "I was diagnosed with cancer and am having a little trouble dealing with it." I tried to sound as nonchalant as possible in an effort to hide the emotions that were bubbling just underneath the surface.

For the first time since we sat down, he turned from this computer to face me. He immediately started asking more questions. However, this time, he wasn't writing down the answers; he kept eye contact with me. The questions were somewhat odd. They were not the normal "oh no, I'm so sorry to hear that, what type of cancer?" type of questions. These were more pointed: "What was your treatment plan? What were the names of the chemotherapies? Did you get really sick? How long did it make you sick? What were your symptoms? How long ago was that? Are you back to normal now?" These types of questions were extremely familiar, but not familiar in the sense that I had been asked by other people. Familiar in the sense that these were the same questions I had after my own diagnosis. I couldn't help but wonder, *Does this guy have cancer?*

Immediately after that thought, he stated that he had just been diagnosed with liver cancer. I could tell he felt a sense of closeness with me, both of us being thrown on the tumultuous roller-coaster ride of a cancer diagnosis. He started telling me things that I had a feeling he had not told many people, if any at all: the deep, dark thoughts that cross your mind after a diagnosis, the ones that are hidden and known only to you.

He told me that since he is going to die, he wants to die on a beautiful beach with a cocktail in his hand, not stuck in the middle of Kansas. When he had told his wife that he was going to pack up and head to a tropical island, she started bawling. He said the tears did not faze him at all; his mind was set. It was his life that was ending; it would be his way. When she told him that she did not want to go to a tropical island for him to die, he replied with, "Okay then, you stay here. I'm going."

While I listened to the therapist continue to admit his secret thoughts and feelings, I felt I was looking in a mirror that showed my own inner turmoil a year ago. I remembered what it was like to want to run away. I remembered feeling like I was going to die and did not care if my family was upset about how I acted or not. If I would have had the funds, I would have wanted to go to some tropical island too. I remembered feeling so alone all I wanted was to be secluded away from everyone I knew—everyone.

He's just saying this now. I remember feeling that way at the very beginning. He will come out of it. After a while, he will realize the tropical island isn't his happy place. His family is his happy place, and he will want to be with them.

As he continued to tell me how the doctor had given the diagnosis, I felt a deep empathy for him. His journey was just starting. He had just gotten thrown into the whirlwind of a cancer diagnosis while I had somehow survived the whirlwind and was now trying to pick myself up off the ground. For the first time since my diagnosis, I felt a sense of gratitude. I was on the opposite side of the spectrum with my journey finally coming to a close. I was past the stage he was at, past the initial shock, past the selfish fear.

He told me that he wished that he could have taken me on for therapy sessions, but he did not feel that would be fair to me because of his upcoming surgery and treatments would be starting soon. He assigned me to a colleague of his, an older gentleman who would be able to help me. As I walked out of the room, I realized that our roles had been ironically reversed. There he was, a middle-aged board-certified psychologist sharing his innermost thoughts with me, a young shattered woman. I was shocked yet somewhat comforted by the realization that everyone is defenseless to the devastation cancer causes.

> *When you go through deep waters, I will be with you. When you go through rivers of difficulty, you will not drown. When you walk through the fire of oppression, you will not be burned up; the flames will not consume you.*
> —Isaiah 43:2 NLT

36

Therapy

I was relieved that the psychiatrist I was assigned to was an older man. I felt that if anyone could handle me, it would have to be someone older with a lot of experience. During the appointment, after a short introduction, he explained, "Now is the time we start seeing cancer patients come in. After the treatments are over and the patient has to start dealing with the mental aspect of having had cancer, it is quite traumatic." That statement made me feel better. He had obviously dealt with cancer patients before, so maybe he would be able to manage my problems.

As the session continued, I admitted to him how horrible I had been acting. I told him how cruel, hateful, resentful, and vicious I had been. It was as though I couldn't control myself. I was completely shocked when he explained how Jesus had gotten angry and overthrew some tables. I was amazed. Not only was my therapist talking about Jesus, but it helped me see that God wasn't sitting there judging me. Rather, he was someone I could relate to.

As the session continued, it surprised me how well the therapist knew what I was feeling. He helped me realize what I was going through was natural. I did not need to be embarrassed or ashamed. For the first time in a long time, I wasn't some freak of nature no one knew what to do with.

Is there finally hope?

He then explained that since I did not have an outlet for my anger, it was all building up, like a pressure cooker. The pressure was building and building until I exploded. The simple way to fix the uncontrollable explosions was to have an outlet for my emotions. He explained that there are many ways of expressing your feelings; the key is to just find a way that is positive. He explained the act of going and beating your neighbor up with a bat was an example of a release of anger, but it was not a good release. I laughed out of shock. The laugh felt good.

The therapist asked if I liked to do any sort of art. My eyes lit up. I loved art. He gave me homework to draw pictures in between our visits. During my return visits, he went through the pictures with me and pointed out things, the first being a tree in a field. He pointed out that the tree was dead with a big hole in it, with everything around it alive and thriving. After hearing him say that, it seemed so obvious that it was clearly a representation of me, yet I somehow hadn't put two and two together. I had simply drawn something that was sitting deep down inside of me, not realizing what it was or why I had drawn it. I was completely blown away that it was a representation of myself—out of place, dead, with a gaping hole while everything around me was not only living but thriving.

How was it possible that my own hand had drawn something with so much meaning, yet I couldn't see the meaning until it was pointed out?

I drew a few more pictures. One was of a spider. I was terrified of spiders, and this one turned out eerily realistic. Another was of a shattered piece of glass. Mostly sketches of broken, sad things. I understood the symbolism of those fairly easily, but there was always something he noticed that I hadn't seen before. Each time he pointed out the hidden symbolism underneath the obvious, I felt a sense of wonder and awe. With each sketch, a piece of my inner self that had been screaming to be let out, to be acknowledged, was finally discovered. With each acknowledgement, I oddly felt a sense of relief.

The drawings continued. There was a sketch of a young girl in a dark alley with broken items lying around her. She was sitting on the dirty, broken ground, leaning against the wall with her head between her knees, arms covering her head. He helped me see that although she was in the shadows, alone, lost, and forgotten, there was a bright sidewalk right beside her. All she had to do was stand up and move into the light. It was there.

"What does that symbolize?" he asked while pointing to a rectangular platform attached to the building above her head. It was bolted to the wall with a metal railing along all open sides of the platform. I sat silent for a few moments, wondering why I had drawn that misplaced platform. *It seems so out of place. It's not even that high. If she were to stand up, she could reach it. Platforms aren't supposed to be that low: people would hit their heads.* Then I realized that there wasn't even a door or ladder to get onto the platform. *How is she supposed to get on it if she wants to?* Had I forgotten something? Was this a mess-up?

I finally admitted, "I don't know," hoping he would fill in the gaps for me as usual. However, he didn't let me press the easy button this time. Instead of giving me the answer, he left it for me to come up with my own conclusion. It sadly wasn't until this very day, where I'm breaking it down in black-and-white, that I finally see what it symbolizes. It had a railing so it would feel safe. It was made of concrete and was bolted into the wall so it was sturdy and stable. It wasn't broken or cracked like the things around it so it was fresh and new. There was no door or ladder so there was a sense of mystery about it. Actually, if I, the broken child, were to simply reach up, I could touch it. It was within my grasp. It was obtainable. If I would just stop looking down at my own mess and look up, I would see it's there. *It* was there the entire time—safe, sturdy, stable, fresh, new, with a hint of mystery, but definitely within my grasp. Tears now fill my eyes as I suddenly realize that my own hand had drawn something that I had been unable to see for so long. And it was Jesus. Jesus had always been there, waiting for me, ready to keep me safe and hold me stable. All I had to do was stop looking at my horrible circumstances and look up. He had been there all along.

> *Trust [confidently] in the Lord forever [He is your fortress, your shield, your banner], For the Lord God is an everlasting Rock [Rock of Ages].*
> —Isaiah 26:4 AMP

37

The Not-So-Gentle Push

It came as quite a shock when Brian casually stated one day, "I found a house."

"What?" *Is he moving out?*

Panic set in. The idea of not having Brian in my life jarred me. For the last year, he had been there, holding me while I cried, bearing the brunt of my anger at the world, and helping me relearn how to laugh again. He was the advocate for change in my life. He wanted me to live a better life, and I had admittedly been quite stubborn when it came to me changing my negative ways. Yet his patience and understanding were things I had come to rely on. It was as if he had been there gently pushing me to find a new, better me. And now he was leaving me? I sat in silence, replaying all the horrible things I had ever done and said to him, knowing him leaving wasn't anything I could hold against him. Yet it hurt and terrified me all at once.

He continued, "I found a house. We move in on Friday."

We? Did he just say we? A sense of relief immediately swept over me. *I'm not losing him. I'm going with him. Wait… I'm going with him? I'm leaving here? My apartment? I can't… I can't do that. This…this… this place is my safe place.*

With the realization that Brian expected me to leave my comfort zone, the one thing that had been a steady constant during the most trying time of my life, I could feel the familiar sense of anger starting to boil deep inside me. *How can he expect me to just change every piece of me overnight? I don't want to leave my home. I can't. I just can't!*

"What do you mean *we* move Friday? That's in three days! I can't just move!" I exclaimed.

He frowned. "Why not?"

I could feel my innermost self screaming the answer so loudly, *Because this is my hole that I have crawled in so deep that I don't think I can come out.*

"I just can't," I snapped. "People don't just move in three days."

"Well, I am. And you're going with me."

Desperate for a reason that didn't expose my most vulnerable self, the truth, my mind started racing for a logical excuse as to why I couldn't make the move.

"Because I have to work Friday! I have work. I can't move Friday. I can't," I said with almost relief. *There's no way around that fact. No moving.*

He cheerfully replied, "Okay, I'll do it." He was obviously happy that my best attempt of an excuse could easily be solved.

My mouth dropped open in astonishment. I did not know what to say. What could I say? *He doesn't understand that I really cannot move. This is my life. This is me. I'll be losing a piece of me—and after all that I've lost already, I literately cannot stand to lose anymore.*

After a few moments of what must have been filled with him contemplating how he would tackle the task of moving everything on his own, he stated with a shrug of his shoulders, "I'm just going to throw everything in the back of the dump truck."

"WHAT!" I envisioned my dishes, my bedding, and my nice clothes all being tossed up over the side of the dump truck, landing in a pile of grease and oil. "You can't do that! What about my dishes? And my *clothes*? Are you just going to throw them in the back of the nasty dump truck? Everything will get ruined!" My eyes were large, waiting for his rebuttal.

"Well, you better start packing what you don't want dirty then," he stated.

Again I was speechless, my mind racing. This was too much to ask of me. Yet he wasn't even asking. He was telling me. He was downright pushing. What happened to the patient, kind man I had grown to love over the last year? Why was he suddenly so forceful with me? Why was he pushing me to do something I couldn't do?

It was obvious that Brian's mind was clearly set. Little did he know, so was mine. *I'm not moving. Ever.*

> *We can make our plans, but the*
> *Lord determines our steps.*
> —Proverbs 16:9 NLT

38

Moving Forward

"I need more boxes. I don't have enough boxes for all of my dishes," I angrily exclaimed while standing over the mix-matched pile of thrift-store dinner plates and bowls that comfortably fit on the small counter. I was well aware of the fact that the large box I was holding would hold all my dishes and then some; however, I was in a mood.

After glancing at the large stack of boxes that took up a large portion of the studio apartment, Brian replied, "You'll make it work." Annoyed with his ability to see through my obvious scheme to cause trouble, I stomped off. I was even more annoyed that he had seen it coming before it even happened, hence the overly crowded pile of packing boxes.

As I slowly wrapped the dishes in newspaper, I couldn't help but wonder why I was treating these dishes as if they were crown jewels. If you really looked at them, they were already scarred and damaged outcasts that had been tossed out in someone's unwanted pile at some point in their existence. As I rubbed my finger along a chipped rim of a plate, I realized those dishes were a resemblance of how I saw myself. I was damaged, cracked, and more than a little rough around the edges. "HANDLE WITH CARE" should have been stamped on my forehead. Just one little mishandle, and I would have easily shattered into a thousand pieces. One wrong move, and I would fall apart. And I was terrified this was that move—literally.

Moving from the apartment that had been the one steady constant during the hardest part of my life wasn't something I felt strong enough to handle. Taking the chance to move forward just to have it all ripped out from underneath me again was a chance I didn't want to take. *I can't go through another letdown. What if I start a new life, and the cancer comes back? I would have to go through all of this all over again—surgery, treatment, exhaustion, pain. Is it best to play it safe and stay in the past with no expectations? How can you fall and get hurt if you're already at the bottom? I don't know what to do. I'm not strong enough for this.*

After just a few hours, the tiny apartment was packed, and the pile of boxes looked as if it had barely been touched. By the time I was off work Friday, we were moved. I felt a deep sense of sorrow driving to the new house instead of the apartment. As I started unpacking things, I realized how very little I actually had. Seeing all of my familiar things spread out in an actual house, exposed in the open spaces, was disheartening. I did not feel like there was enough of me to fill that house. It was empty and scattered—and so was I.

Although I didn't physically move the items during the move, the stress of it all suddenly made me feel completely exhausted. The effects of the chemotherapy were still causing havoc on my body. When I was tired, I was dead tired. I lay down on the bare mattress that was on the floor and slept for three hours.

When I woke, it was time to go meet the landlord of my old apartment for a final walk-through. As I handed over my apartment key, I watched, in what seemed to be slow motion, as the cancer-ribbon-shaped key was being pulled out of my hand. I stood in silence, staring at my fingers, as the symbolism nearly knocked me off my feet. Not only was I handing over the key to my apartment, I was literally letting go of cancer itself. I surprised myself as I realized I was grasping harder to the key he was trying to take from my hand in a desperate attempt to hang on. He shot me a confused glance. We stood there for a moment, awkwardly holding the key between the two of us. I suddenly let go. I turned without saying a word and headed for the exit. I felt my breath get caught in my throat as I shut the door on the past.

Tears started streaming down my face as I quickly rushed to my car. On the drive back to the new house, I started sobbing so uncontrollably that I had to pull over into a parking lot to try to gather myself. The future was such a scary possibility. What had happened to me wasn't something I could just move past; it was part of who I was now. It always would be. It had changed me forever. As tragic as what had happened to me was, I still didn't want to leave that space, that time period, that life. I felt I was leaving a piece of myself behind. As I sat there bawling, I couldn't help but to ask myself, *Am I really ready to let go? Am I really ready to take that first step toward a future I was told I would never have—only to be dragged back through all of this again? Am I that brave?*

After probably a good half hour, my sobbing subsided. I couldn't stay in that parking lot forever. Nor could I stay in the past. It was time. Time to let go. As much as I didn't want to, time was up. Somehow through the tears and fear, I put my car into drive and started moving forward toward an unknown future.

I know the Lord is always with me. I will not be shaken, for he is right beside me.
—Psalm 16:8 NLT

39

The True Beginning

After the move, a few more therapy appointments came and went. I started to get this feeling that the therapy sessions, as helpful as they were, had become somewhat repetitive. I felt an inner urge for something more. I just couldn't quite put my finger on what that was or where to find it. Then the therapist suggested I start reading the Bible. By this time, he had figured out I had no idea what he was talking about with his many Bible references. He explained that most people start with Matthew, Luke, and John to learn about Jesus and his life of ministry. He suggested I start with John.

So I did. I was truly amazed to see so many instances of healing. From what I gathered from the little I had read, that's what took up most of Jesus's time: healing the sick. It must have been important to him. I was mind-blown. I'm not sure what I expected Jesus to do on a daily basis, but I didn't expect him to be traveling among the poor, sickly sinners and extending grace toward them. He really went out of his way to let the people know how much he wanted them healed, healthy, and whole.

My pictures started to shift. I drew a picture of a girl standing on a grassy field in a cute dress in front of a sunset. Her arms were stretched out wide, upward, and birds were flying happily above her toward the sun. It gave me a sense of breaking free—freedom. Another drawing was of a girl on a swing underneath a luscious tree in front of a pretty sunset on a grassy hilltop. It symbolized that life can be enjoyable and hinted toward my desire to be happy again. I drew another image of a girl being lifted up by a balloon into a bright, cheery sky. It represented me going places, following my dreams, having a future.

With each drawing, I felt as though I was putting a piece of myself onto the paper. The process was still translating something I wasn't quite able to put into words. Then, oddly, I felt a desire to start writing. The therapist explained why that made sense. The drawings brought out feelings that I hadn't been able to understand, let alone define with words. Once those basic feelings were brought into the light, I needed to release more in a more controlled manner. It only made sense to move to the next step—writing.

Early on in the process of being diagnosed, I had started keeping a journal. Nothing big and definitely not routine. Just a few things here and there, mainly complaints and fears. The urge to write more continued to grow. I thought about it often, and you could say I felt a tinge of excitement. I couldn't remember the last time I was excited about something. Yet the idea of handwriting the whole mess of what had happened in detail seemed like a chore. The urge grew even stronger, so much so that I started to wonder if it wasn't God trying to tell me to write my story. I couldn't help but remember that odd encounter with the woman at the library who I thought could have been my Aunt Gayle.

She distinctly told me, "Your story is going to inspire so many people." Can it be true? Can this be the beginning of something? The true beginning of why I was put through hell and back? Or am I just overthinking this? Let's face it, that was probably some crazy old lady rambling.

I couldn't help but wonder, *But what if...*

I decided to put it in God's hands. If he wanted me to actually write, if this urge was from him, if that old batty lady really wasn't crazy after all, then he would give me a sign—surely. I mean, come on, he brought people back from the dead, turned water into wine, and parted the red seas. Surely if he really wanted me to do this, he would do this one thing for me. So as I lay in bed, I prayed, *God, if this really is you telling me this, if you really do want me to write my story, please give me a laptop to write it on.*

My jaw hit the floor the very next day when Brian walked in the front door with a laptop under his arm. "Look what I traded Guillermo!" he happily said as he sat it on the coffee table directly in front of me.

I sat, silent, eyes large, staring at the laptop in disbelief. I had never experienced anything like this before. I couldn't believe my eyes.

"What's wrong?" he asked.

"Where did you get that?" I asked while still staring at the laptop.

"I traded those old rims for it. Thought, heck, why not? I thought you might use it, but if not, that's fine. I'll just trade it for something else."

I started crying. This was a clear and definite answer to the prayer the night before. No mistaking that.

God wants me to write my story. God *wants me to write my story. God wants* ME *to write* MY *story. He went out of his way for* me. *Little ole me. God just spoke to me. He heard me. He sees me. He cares. Maybe there really is a reason I went through all that I have gone through. Is this it? Is this the beginning of something bigger?*

Brian interrupted my epiphany with, "What's going on?" His voice was raised.

I suddenly realized that he must have thought I was upset that he brought a laptop home. I quickly started rambling through the tears. After my explanation of what I had prayed just the night before and why, we both sat in silence, staring at the laptop. We were both blown away. There was no way this was a coincidence. Not this one. This was a sign that God *did* want me to begin writing my story. I had an even stronger feeling that it was for a reason larger than myself.

Writing this story was hard. The hardest thing I've ever done. However, I was not alone. With each and every long night filled with heart-throbbing tears, I felt the presence of the Lord pushing me to go forward. Piece by piece, this story slowly came together, each chapter with its own special revelations. I had no idea while writing this that I would find healing. The simple act of writing down the events that had happened opened the door for me to start processing. Categorizing the chaos brought structure, and through that structure, I was able to acknowledge and simply allow all the emotions to run their course. This book brought closure to the long and weary story so that God could start my true beginning. My new life. The new me.

> *Now stand here and see the great
> thing the Lord is about to do.*
> —1 Samuel 12:16 NLT

40

The Reason

This book was written in hopes of finding you—the lost, the broken, the shaken. You're not alone. I, along with a large amount of other strong survivors, have witnessed the devastation on our loved one's faces when they heard the news. We too have spent countless nights sobbing in corners. We too have envisioned our own funerals. We get it. I get it. And that's why I have kept coming back to finish this book, year after year (nine years to be exact). To give hope—to you. Yes, you.

But there is even bigger news in this short chapter: you're not only *my* reason, but you're God's reason too.

You see, God wants to bless you. He wants to heal you. He wants to keep you safe. He wants you happy. All you have to do is just believe. Believe that the healing is already yours through the stripes of Jesus. Believe that God loves you so very much that he gave his Son at the cross for *you*. Yes, you. And this is the good news that I hope you hear and take in. This all is for you. This book is for you. Jesus is for you. Healing is for you. You are the reason.

And his name will be the hope of all the world.
—Matthew 12:21 NLT

About the Author

After graduating with a bachelor's degree in elementary education, Jessica pursued a career teaching preschool to low-income families in order to touch lives that were similar to her own childhood. She worked there for several years before, during, and after her cancer diagnosis. She eventually left the full-time job on a leap of faith and is now able to pursue her love of arts while selling her handmade items.

Whether it's watching a movie with her husband, eating her favorite dessert (wedding cake), or reading her Bible, she tries to make the most of each moment. In her opinion, God has blessed her with a second chance, and she doesn't want to waste it.

CPSIA information can be obtained
at www.ICGtesting.com
Printed in the USA
BVHW030806130123
655992BV00022B/364